The Oral-Facial Therapy Exercise Book
2021 Edition

by Debra C. Gangale CCC/slp

Illustrations by Deborah Curzon Crocker
Cover Design and Editing by Beverly Lorenc

MCRO Publishing
Prior editions published by Pro-Ed, Inc. and LinguiSystems, Inc.

Copyright © 2021

All products are copyrighted to protect the fine work of the author. You may copy the exercises, forms, and charts only as needed for your own use with clients. Any other reproduction or distribution of the pages in this book is prohibited, including copying the entire book to use as another primary source or "master" copy.

Skill	Ages
■ oral motor	■ elementary through adult

This book and recommendations from this book are intended for use with guidance and instruction of a skilled oral-facial professional.
These professionals may include:

- Dentist
- Orthodontist
- Speech Language Pathologist

Asha.org

The American Speech and Hearing Association is the national professional, scientific, and credentialing association for audiologists; speech-language pathologists; speech, language, and hearing scientists; audiology and speech-language pathology support personnel; and students. Contacting ASHA can locate a licensed Speech language pathologist in your area.

Table of Contents

Introduction 7
Motivating the Client 9
Suggestions for Performing and Scheduling Exercises 10
Universal Precautions 11
Chapter 1: Breathing and Visualization 12
Chapter 2: Communication 26
Chapter 3: Posture and Stretches 32
Chapter 4: Drooling Management 39
Chapter 5: Stimulation Therapy 42
Chapter 6: Neck Exercises 50
Chapter 7: Voice Exercises 57
Chapter 8: Cheek Exercises 76
Chapter 9: Jaw Exercises 85
Chapter 10: Lip Exercises 98
Chapter 11: Tongue Exercises 126
Chapter 12: Nasal Exercises 149
Chapter 13: Ear Exercises 153
Assessments, Evaluations and Forms 157
    Referral Sheet 158
    Request for Release of Medical Records 159
    Oral-Facial Swallowing Evaluation and Rating Scale 160
    Oral-Facial Function Evaluation 165
    Visual Facial Charting 170
    Client Care Plan 171
    Neurological Daily Status Update 172
    Speech-Language Pathology Status Update 175
    Sample Phonation Chart 176
    Phonation Chart 177
    Oral Motor Exercise Chart - Lips 178
    Oral Motor Exercise Chart - Tongue 179
    Rancho Levels of Cognitive Function 180
    Standardized Speech Samples 181
    Grandfather Passage 182
    The Wish Passage 183
    Affirmation of Composure and Harmony 184

Table of Contents, continued

Front View of Musculature 185
Back View of Musculature 186
References 187

Foreward

All treatments should be part of the treatment plan which is signed and approved by the individual's primary physician. If the individual does not show pain relief or increase in function, it is best to suggest another type of intervention such as physical therapy, occupational therapy, advanced myofascial therapy, neuromuscular massage intervention, counseling, or other pain management strategies referred by the physician.

Disclaimer

The Oral Facial Therapy Exercise Book: 2021 Edition is a resource book to assist you in developing a therapy program for individuals with oral-facial disorders. Please remember that aspiration can occur even with strict adherence to proper positioning and precautions. This book may accompany the individual home for independent use. It is best used with the supervision of a licensed speech-language pathologist, occupational therapist, or physical therapist. The Author and the publisher assume no responsibility for the inaccurate interpretation or application of the theories, procedures, and techniques presented in this book.

Introduction

The Oral-Facial Therapy Exercise Book: 2021 Edition includes everything you'll need to evaluate a client with oral-facial disorders and to implement a therapy program. This comprehensive listing of interventions and exercises provides you with a wide variety of tools to meet your client's needs. The large type and clear line illustrations make the simple exercises ideal to reproduce for clients.

It's important to consider each client individually when establishing a remediation program. Each situation brings a unique set of needs and may require ongoing modifications to the number of therapy sessions per week, short-term and long-term goals, and overall progress. The exercises in this book will benefit clients with a variety of oral-facial disorders including those associated with:

- cerebral palsy
- Parkinson's disease
- mental retardation
- head trauma
- cranio-facial anomalies
- Bell's palsy

Exercises and intervention goals may be as follows and are listed per exercise:

- balance flaccid and tense musculature
- inhibit and facilitate movement
- relax and focus the client
- stimulate flaccid muscle tissue
- decrease tactile defensiveness
- increase productive usage of musculature for deglutition, articulation, and voicing
- decrease pain response
- improve vocal quality and vocal projection
- improve attention span
- improve communication
- improve energy awareness
- strengthen client, clinician, family, and support staff communication in rehabilitation
- increase oral awareness
- develop more precise oral movements for eating and drinking
- increase speech intelligibility through phrasing or motor planning

The goal of *The Oral-Facial Therapy Exercise Book: 2020 Edition* is to allow the individual to work with you to manage a program of recovery that is all inclusive to the individual. This book is intended for use with inpatients, outpatients, home healthcare, or as a take-home workbook for clients.

Introduction, continued

You'll notice that some of the exercises are written to you, the speech-language pathologist (SLP), and some are written directly to the client. This is because many of the exercises can be performed directly by the client or with assistance from an SLP or aide. Become familiar with each page so that you are better able to locate the intervention that specifically fits your needs for rehabilitation.

An oral-motor team that supports attainment of the client's oral-motor goals is vital to success. The ideal situation is to include all people who interact with the individual for his overall health and recovery. Use the members of the team on a regular basis for support, instruction, and care plan development. Team members may include:

- patient

- family members

- physicians – primary physician or any other M.D. directly or indirectly related to patient recovery (e.g., otolaryngologist [Ear, Nose, and Throat specialist])

- nurses

- speech-language pathologist (SLP) – certified individual trained to develop and rehabilitate communication, voice, and swallowing

- occupational therapist (OT) – certified individual trained to develop and rehabilitate gross, fine, and perceptual motor functions for living and vocational skills

- physical therapist (PT) – certified individual trained to rehabilitate overall skeletal-muscular strength and range of motion

- audiologist – certified individual trained to test and treat hearing-related difficulties

- neuromuscular massage therapist – specialist in all forms of deep tissue work, myofascial release, integrative body therapy, and/or experience with medical conditions

- augmentative communication specialist – may be an SLP who will develop an alternate means of communication (e.g., sign language, communication board, picture cards, letter board). Augmentative communication relieves the stress of communication while regaining speech intelligibility during oral-motor therapy.

- social worker

Motivating the Client

Throughout therapy, it is important to gauge the motivation of the individual and his desire to be helped. Passive interventions such as massage, acupressure, and sensory stimulation are good ways to help an individual test the water. Many times an individual is fearful of hurting himself when stretching or when doing a repetitive movement. Success at lower levels can prove to a client that it is safe to move forward.

Begin by giving the individual a mix of exercises. Include more difficult exercises with easy or achieved motor movements. This will assure follow-through and continued participation. Then incrementally move toward greater proficiency, strength, and function of movement. Slowly attained, small gains are better than fast and constant failures. Setting easy, attainable goals builds confidence, patience, and endurance for later goals that will be more challenging.

Positive Affirmations

Some clients may be motivated through the use of positive affirmations. Affirmations are positive statements concerning ways we want to think, feel, and behave. They help paint a mental picture of what a person wants to achieve. When a person gives attention to a particular goal, more energy is focused on it. The more something is desired, the more likely it is to be realized. Using positive affirmations during therapy can help a client focus on the goal he is trying to achieve.

When starting an exercise, explain the goal to the client. For example, you might say, "We're going to work on moving your tongue tip up. This will help you swallow more efficiently. We're going to use this tongue depressor for you to push against. It will give your tongue resistance and make it strong. The goal is to get your tongue tip to go up. Let me show you what that looks like."

Then help the client restate the goal using positive affirmations. For example, the client might say, "I can move my tongue tip up. I can push against the tongue depressor. I can make my tongue strong. I can swallow more efficiently." If needed, shorten the affirmation to "I can make my tongue strong," or "I can swallow better."

You might want to write the affirmations on an index card for the client. If the client cannot express himself verbally, it will serve as a positive mental note to practice. Encourage the client to repeat the affirmation(s) as often as needed.

Suggestions for Performing and Scheduling Exercises

When performing exercises on a client, it's important to first touch him on the shoulder or arm to acquaint him with the texture and pressure of your hand. This will also reduce a startle reflex which can occur if you begin by directly touching the client's face.

As the exercises are performed, tell the client what your next move will be and what to expect. Many patients show tactile defensiveness due to lack of touch (e.g., neglected, serious illness) or fear that the exercise might inflict pain.

The exercises can be performed one to five times per day – seven days a week. It's important to develop a program for the client that designates which exercises to do, the number of repetitions per exercise, and the number of times per day. If tolerated, the average routine is 10 repetitions per exercise, three or four times per day unless otherwise noted. The best results will occur with daily exercise. You'll often find clients who enjoy exercising so much, they far exceed the prescribed number of exercises.

If any exercise causes pain, have the client try it again using a shorter range of motion and less muscular effort. A change in how the exercise is being performed may relieve the discomfort. Minor discomfort can be expected in the beginning because the client's muscle groups may be atrophied, very weak, and/or unaccustomed to movement. Generally, clients find the exercises to be soothing. The exercises also tend to relieve the discomfort associated with restricted range of motion and weak musculature.

When the client is performing the exercises for the first time, it's best to eliminate any distractions like the radio or competing conversations. Once the client is familiar with the exercises, soft background music can be relaxing.

Universal Precautions

Universal precautions refer to the laws set in place to maintain healthy safe interactions with any individual in any setting. These precautions are usually available at the facility or through your employer. It is imperative that they are followed. Basically for oral-motor interventions, it is advised:

- wash hands between each client

- wear a new set of gloves for each client

- avoid touching yourself when wearing the gloves as they may have been in or around the client's mouth or an open wound

- wash and disinfect all materials between clients

- use tongue depressors, lemon swabs, bite blocks, Chewy Tubes, laryngeal mirrors, and Toothettes for one client only and dispose after use

Remember that some individuals may be allergic to latex, tape (e.g., adhesive tape, therapy tape), or plastic. Check with the nurse, the family, and/or the individual before using them or any other new materials.

Inquire before using any materials, foods or liquids that the individual may be allergic to. Check to see if the individual has any allergies to any substances before working with any exercises, materials, food and/or liquids. Consult with the parent, physician, therapist, teacher, individual and review all files and charts that may indicate any allergies.

Chapter 1:
Breathing and Visualization

> "It has been known for centuries that it is possible to induce profound changes in body, mind, and spirit by techniques which involve breathing." — Stanislav Grof

"How could I have forgotten how to breathe?"

This is the most common remark made by individuals experiencing difficulties with inadequate breath support or improper breath usage. The ability to breathe in (inhalation) and out (exhalation) for sound (phonation), tone (resonation), and speech (articulation) is taken for granted. The individual experiencing difficulties might:

- use short breaths

- shallow breaths

- hold breath while attempting phonation and word production

- exhaust air supply before the words are spoken and speak on residual air

- fail to replenish air supply and trail off voice followed by a large, strained, audible inhalation

- mouth words only with little or no attempt at coordinating speech on a voice exhalation

Exercises to provide adequate respiration are key to any program for relaxation, phonation, and/or articulation. The client learns to produce a breathing pattern of inhalation and exhalation for rest breathing and for speech. The amount of air necessary for rest breathing is the same amount as is required for speech.

Using the diagram on the next page, describe the Circular Breathing technique to the client. Explain how the technique will help her:

- visualize the breathing cycle

- monitor rate and length of inhalation and exhalation

- reinforce facial, neck, and body relaxation through imagery

The Oral-Facial Therapy Exercise Book
2021 Edition

Chapter 1, *continued*

- establish rhythm to breathing cycle

- learn to lower breathing pattern to abdominal-diaphragmatic without confusing details or explanations

- voice upon exhalation using gentle onset of phonation

- replenish air based on kinesthetic (feeling the need for new air supply) approach

Circular Breathing without Voicing

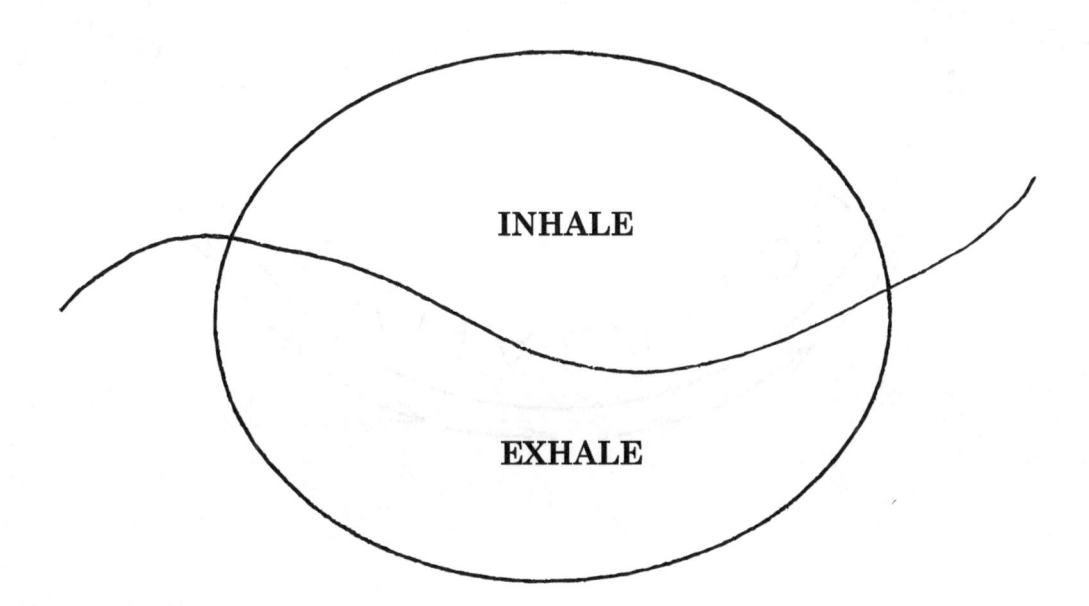

INHALE

EXHALE

Circular breathing is a simple way to help relax and focus clients. By establishing a slow, relaxed rhythm for inhalation and exhalation, it can help clients improve voicing and articulation. It also releases overall body tensions and can help reduce frustrations when learning a new task. This technique can also be used to slow down or speed up a client's energy level.

This breathing technique is effective for patients with Parkinson's disease, Alzheimer's disease, cerebral palsy, multiple sclerosis, and Amyotrophic Lateral Sclerosis (ALS) as well as patients who have had head injuries (e.g., cerebral vascular accident [CVA]).

Chapter 1, *continued*

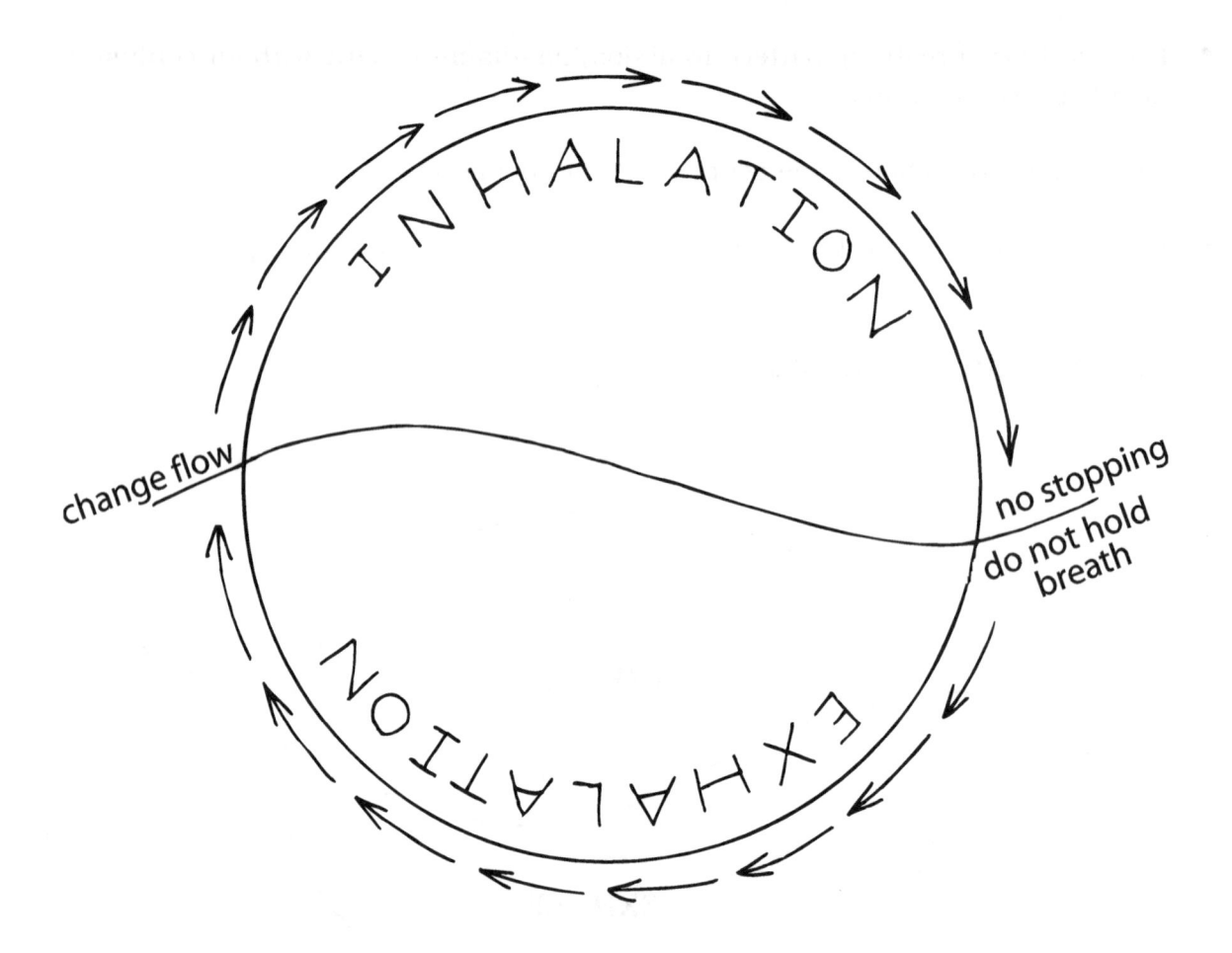

[Diagram of a circle labeled INHALATION on top half and EXHALATION on bottom half, with arrows showing flow. Labels: "change flow" on the left, "no stopping, do not hold breath" on the right.]

- Relax face, head, neck, shoulders, and body.
- Make slow, full inhalation/exhalation while tracing the diagram with your finger.
- Inhale slowly, with full inhalation on the upper half of the circle.
- Exhale slowly, effortlessly on the bottom half of the circle.
- Establish a slow, relaxed rhythm as you inhale and exhale.
- Breathe air in and down as if into the stomach when inhaling.

Chapter 1, *continued*

Imagery

The following descriptions can be paraphrased or read to clients to further help them visualize the Circular Breathing technique. Take the time to demonstrate how it is done properly. Repeat information as needed.

> **Inhalation:** Use a slow, quiet, unforced full breath. Imagine slowly filling your stomach with air. Don't overfill it, just let the air flow into your stomach. As you trace the diagram, maintain a slow, even inhalation. You want your inhalation to last as you trace the top half of the circle. If you hear noise when you inhale, it means there's some stress or tension. Breathe through your nose with your mouth closed. Concentrate on quiet inhalation. If you can still hear your own breath, continue by inhaling more slowly.
>
> **Change Flow:** Exhaling the air should be easy. Just let the air fall out. Concentrate on feeling the sensation of air moving slowly, without effort, out of your nose. The flow of air should never stop. Your index finger should continue tracing the circle without stopping, slowing, or speeding up. Relax into an even, rhythmic flow around the circle.
>
> **Exhalation:** As you exhale, completely let all of your muscle effort go. If it helps, silently count to 10 or say the word *exhale* or *release* as you exhale.
>
> **Relaxation:** It's important to relax as you practice your breathing. Start by releasing your facial muscles and then your jaw muscles. As you exhale and trace the diagram, concentrate on relaxing your neck, shoulders, arms, and hands. Then relax your stomach, buttocks, legs, and feet. Think about how relaxed your body feels while your eyes are closed. Trace the diagram in your mind, feeling your stomach fill as you inhale and empty as you exhale.

Suggested practice is 20 times around the diagram, five times daily or when physically and/or emotionally stressed.

Circular Breathing with Hum

The transition to voicing can produce unwanted habitual glottal attacks or improper breathing patterns of holding the breath while voicing. This will cause the client to attempt to speak using an insufficient residual air supply. The transition from exhale-only breathing to exhaling while humming will transfer optimal breathing patterns to voicing.

Recommended practice is 10 times around the diagram, five times daily. This exercise will help your client control her breathing as she learns to coordinate words and phrases with air flow.

Chapter 1, *continued*

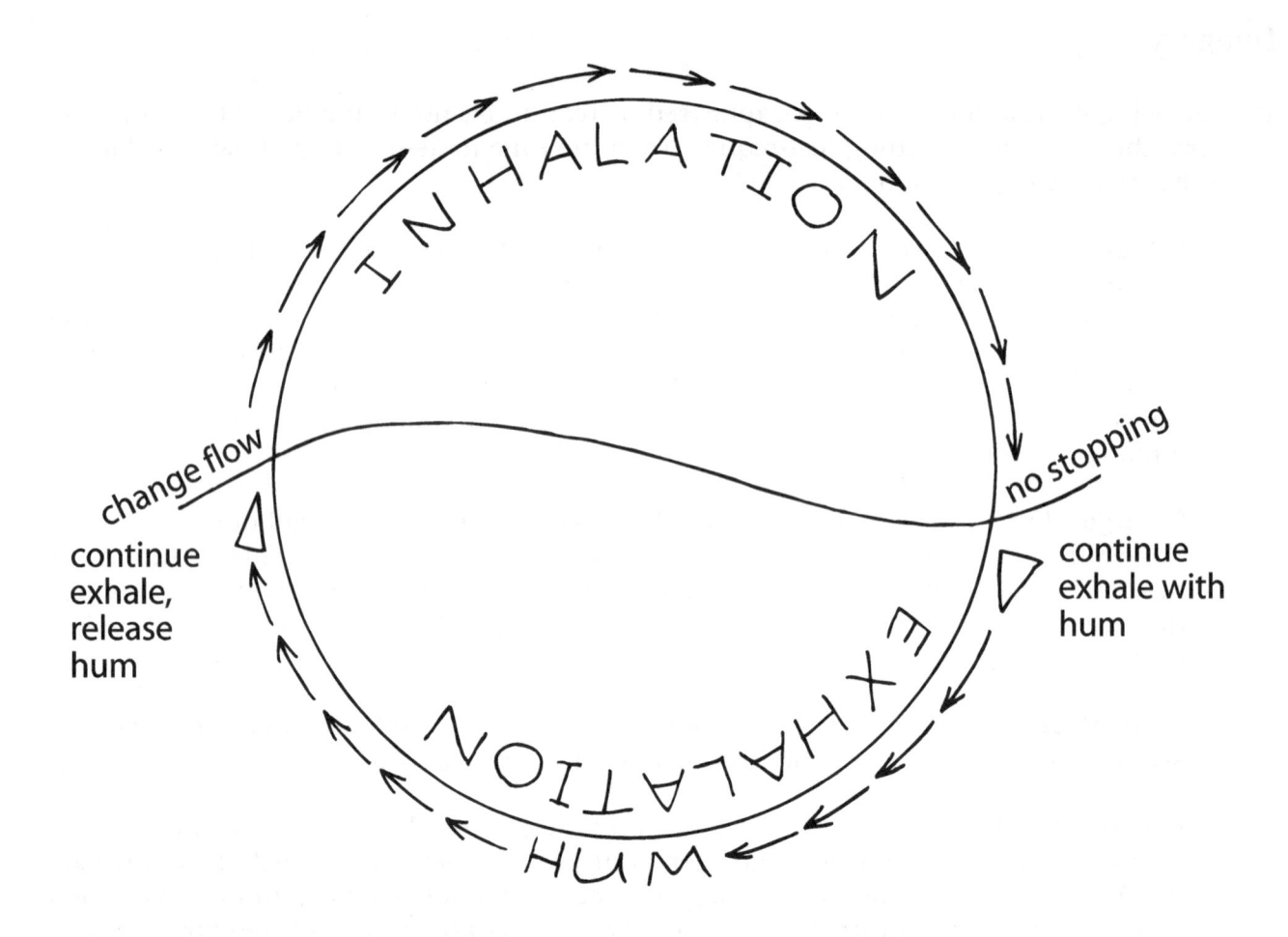

Diagram: Circular breathing cycle showing INHALATION (top half) and EXHALATION HUM (bottom half), with labels "change flow — continue exhale, release hum" on the left and "no stopping — continue exhale with hum" on the right.

Inhalation: This is the same as in Circular Breathing without Voicing. Slowly and quietly inhale as you fill your stomach with air. Trace your index finger around the circle to indicate your place in inhalation.

Change Flow: Do this the same as in Circular Breathing without Voicing. Release into a relaxed, unforced, light, and effortless flow without stopping.

Exhalation: Initiate sound shortly after you begin to exhale. It requires little muscular effort. Keep the same Circular Breathing rhythm going with no change in air pressure, muscular effort, or rate. Begin humming quietly, slowly, and effortlessly. Feel the sensation in the back of your nose as the vibration from the hum fills your nasal cavity. Stop humming shortly before your index finger approaches the change flow indicator. Continue exhaling until you reach the change flow indicator. Then repeat the cycle on the diagram.

The hum should be relaxing. Trace the diagram with your index finger, establishing a rhythm. When the change flow and the phonation are initiated without stopping, close your eyes and concentrate on relaxing your face, neck, and shoulders. Continue relaxing the rest of your body with each hum.

The Oral-Facial Therapy Exercise Book
2021 Edition

Chapter 1, continued

Building on the Circular Breathing with Hum

1. After the client demonstrates proficiency at the hum level, progress during the next session to /h/ phoneme-initiated syllables:

   he   hi   ho   ha   hih   huh   hoo

   Ask the client to elongate the vowel sound like a sigh as she exhales.

2. Continue with /h/-initiated one-syllable words such as:

he	hill	hair	ham	whose
hum	hi	hot	help	hole
his	hoop	hope	head	hear
him	who	home	hall	heat

3. Progress to other phoneme-initiated, one-syllable words or continue to /h/-initiated bisyllabic words or phrases. As new phoneme-initiated syllables and multisyllabic words are introduced, return to the Circular Breathing with Hum to review and maintain the optimal flow of air.

   Note: The phonemes /b, p, t, d, k, g/ and the vowel sounds *oh, eye, ah, ay* may increase muscular involvement, interrupt exhalation, and decrease optimal voice production. If so, teach each phonological group (i.e., back phonemes /k, g/ or plosive phonemes /p, b, t, d/) separately with vowel elongation on exhalation.

4. Refer to Box Speech in Chapter 8 to teach the client to phrase and replenish air supply at the sentence level.

Muscle Relaxation

Muscle rigidity is one factor associated with many disorders and diseases, such as Parkinson's disease. This rigidity can be caused by improper positioning, stress, and muscle fatigue. In clients who are mild to moderately affected, relaxation exercises can be useful in reducing muscle rigidity. The following exercise is excellent for body orientation as well as for relaxation.

To begin, ask the client to make two fists, stiffening her hands and arms. Have the client hold the tense muscles for five seconds. Follow this with deep relaxation of the same muscles. Repeat with the same muscle group three times. Allow at least five seconds of relaxation between each clench.

Continue the exercise with the neck, jaw, stomach, back, legs, and feet, first tensing and then relaxing each muscle group.

Deep Full Breath

This exercise helps individuals learn (or relearn) how to take a deep, full breath.

A spontaneous breath that is full and free helps establish a flexible center (e.g., soft, responsive neck, vocal folds, rib cage, and thoracic area) and releases the vocal cords and neck for resonant voicing. Clavicular breathing and/or breathing high in the upper chest can interfere with voicing, causing audible inhalations and subsequent strain to the vocal folds. Inhaling so the breath goes into the lower chest and diaphragm may help to decrease tension in the jaw, neck, face, and shoulders. It gives the ribs an inner stretch to improve overall body relaxation and well-being. Inhaling deeply so the air goes into the lower chest and diaphragm creates a larger breath capacity which, in turn, increases vocal intensity (loudness).

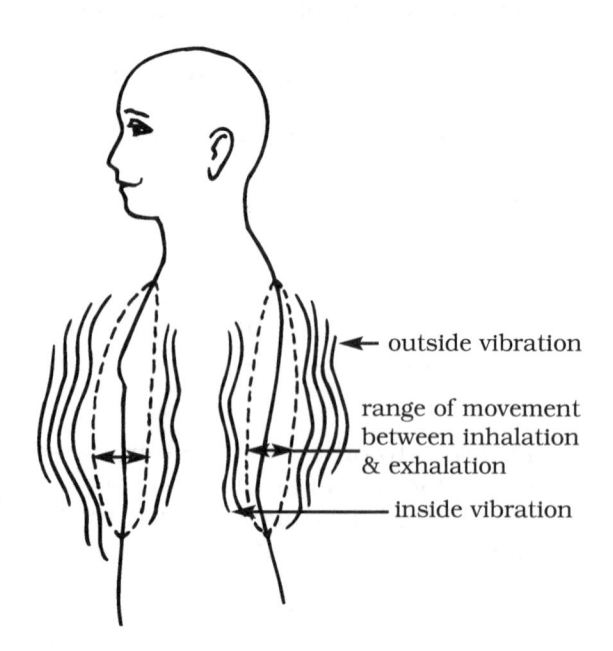

This exercise is especially useful with clients with Parkinson's disease as their breath tends to become shallow and restricted. Increasing breath volume can have a direct affect on attention span, concentration, and mood stabilization.

The result of learning this exercise is body and mind centering. An alert, relaxed, and energized individual can offer more to her own recovery process. Her input and feedback can help you plan therapy and revise goals.

Say to the client:

"As you inhale, your breath expands and vibrates throughout your entire rib cage. As you exhale, your breath spontaneously lets go without any pushing or assistance from a forced or deliberate squeeze of your stomach. No effort is required to exhale. Do not squeeze your chest. Simply inhale and then let go of the air. Just let it fall out. Let your body decide when it is time to bring a fresh inhalation back into your lower chest.

"Sometimes it's useful to think about filling your belly with air and letting it go. Then take another breath and fill your belly and your pelvic area with air. Let it go. Finally fill your belly, pelvic area, and legs and feet with air and let it go. This visualization will deepen and expand your breath. Keep yourself focused as you breathe in lower and lower and then exhale by merely letting go."

Supine Breath Expansion

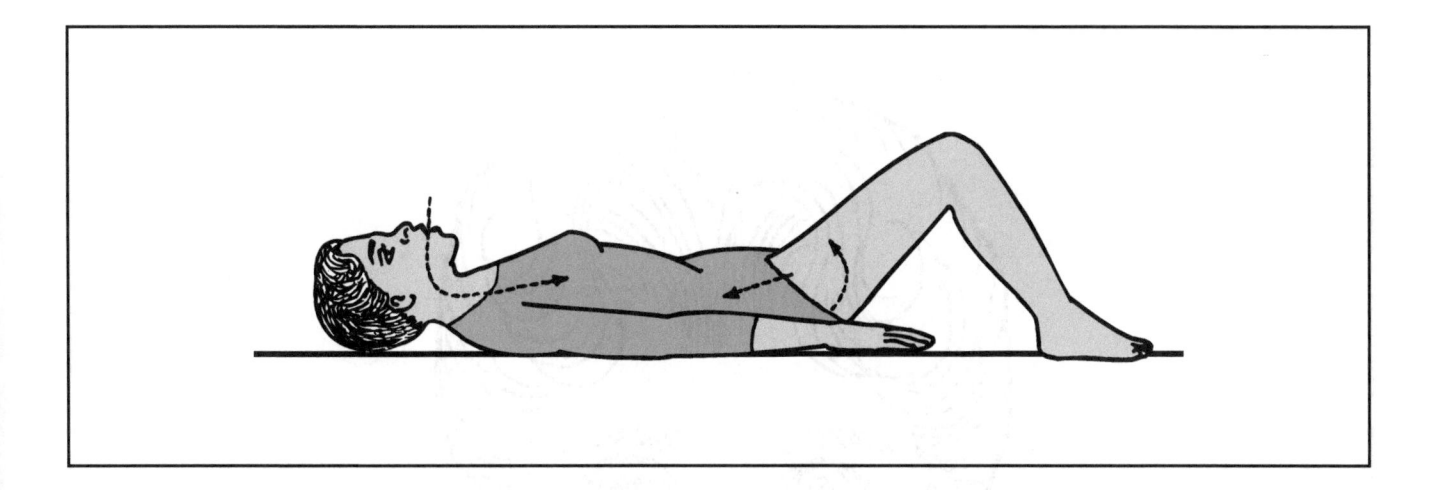

Chapter 1, continued

1. Lie relaxed. Make sure your back and neck are comfortable. Bend your knees naturally, place a pillow under your knees, or adjust yourself to what feels comfortable.

2. Inhale. Allow the air to flow into your chest. Exhale.

3. Inhale again, but now allow the air to flow through your chest into your abdomen. Exhale.

4. Now inhale so the air feels like it is filling your chest, abdomen, and pelvis. Exhale.

5. Continue breathing in and out slowly and fully. Be sure the air fills your abdomen and pelvis. Exhale naturally. Repeat 10 to 15 times.

There is no goal to achieve here except a feeling of well-being so relax, breathe, and expand!

> Breath work changes who we are, our attitude, and our view of ourselves. It also allows us to be and achieve far more than our mental self-imposed limitations.

Rise and Shine Stimulating Breath Exercise

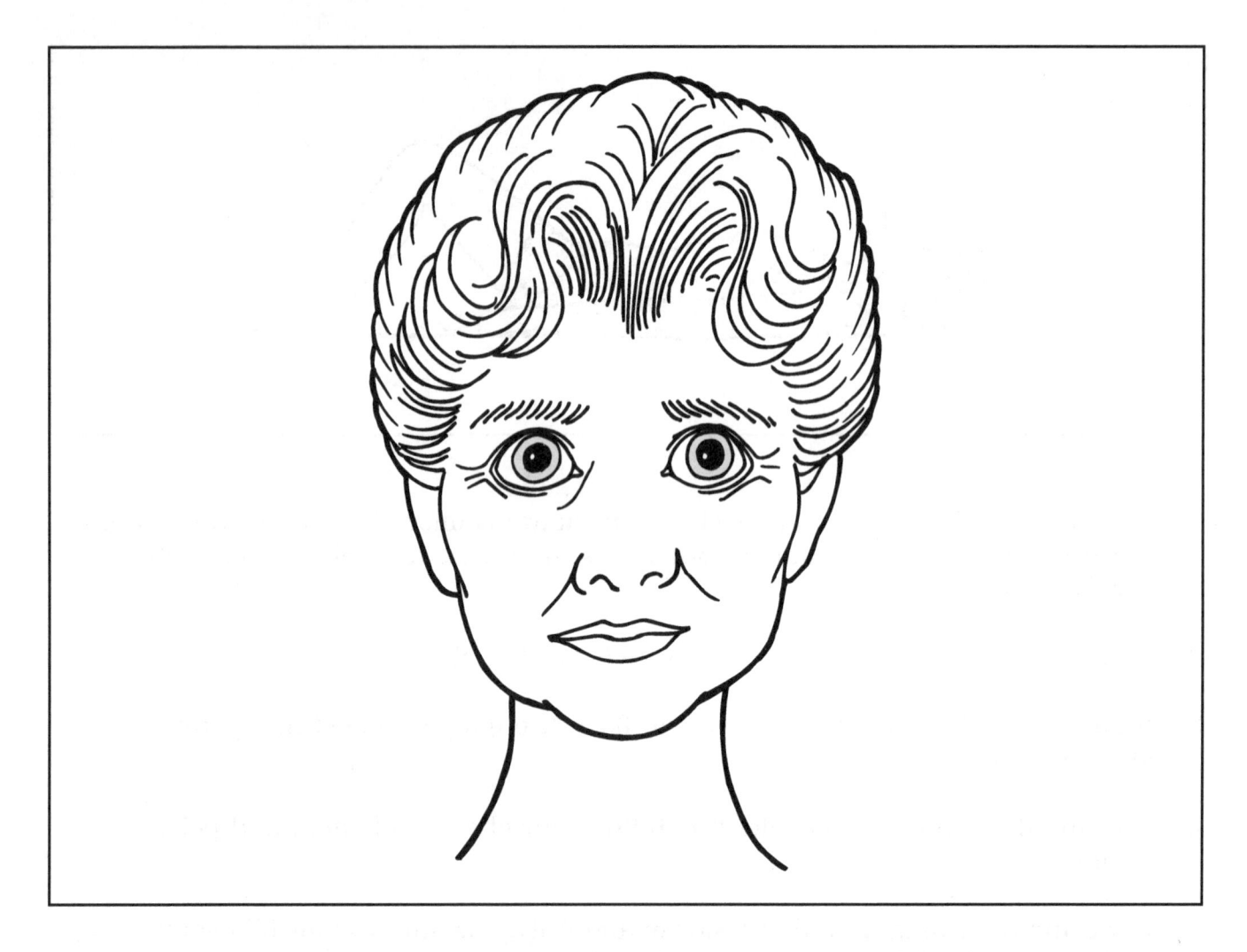

Open your eyes very, very wide. Force your eyeballs to open wide (bug-eye) and inhale with all of your might. Then let out all of your air and relax your eyes. Repeat 5 times.

Benefit

○ prepares for the interventions and exercises that follow

Chapter 1, continued

Visualization

Visualization is the process of letting the mind and body act together through guided imagery. Spoken words, written words, and/or pictures can enhance a person's ability to perform an exercise. Often when a client visualizes outcomes or uses a symbol to represent the achieved goal, it can increase the likelihood of success.

Before the visualization begins, make sure the client is comfortable. Have the client close her eyes.

During the visualization, use a nice tone of voice (e.g., soothing, appropriate loudness). Speak slowly so the client can sense and visualize the meditation. As you talk, remember to breathe evenly. Release any tensions you feel with a deep breath.

At the end, provide time for silent reflection. Ask the client to open her eyes when she is ready. As she opens her eyes, make eye contact and smile. Ask the client if she wishes to talk or write about the experience. You might want to establish an anchor word or symbol (e.g., cross [faith], star [focus], sky [expansion], tree [steadiness]) to help the client describe the feeling or awareness from the visualization. You can then use that word or symbol later to quickly center the client.

To get you started, three visualizations are on the following pages. These visualizations can be performed on the same day or on different days, and they may be performed in any order. They are very effective when taught in order as Body Breathing helps with increasing inhalation, the Cleansing Breath works to release the exhalation, and Breath Awareness brings inhalation and exhalation together.

1. Body Breathing: This is a good starter breath visualization to gain focus and increase attention span. It is very relaxing.

2. Cleansing Breath: This visualization helps to release tension, anxiety, and feelings of tightness. It provides renewed energy.

3. Breath Awareness: This visualization is a very effective breath visualization to use with the Circular breathing exercises in Chapter 1.

Body Breathing

"Breathe in and out through your nose and feel, sense, or imagine that with every inhalation, you can draw energy in and through the entire surface of your body. Simply imagine that each slow, deep, inhaled breath is drawing energy in through each cell of your body; that the whole outer surface of your skin opens to and receives energy with each deep, inhaled breath; and, as you listen, you feel, sense, or imagine that with every exhalation, you radiate energy outward, like a glowing light or a burning flame. With every exhalation, the entire surface of your body releases and radiates energy. Continue breathing in through your skin and radiating out through your skin for a few more minutes."

Cleansing Breath

"Breathe in through your nose and with each inhale, sense that the air is coming in through the soles of your feet. Then breathe in as if you have to pull the air up through your feet, ankles, legs, hips, and torso until you blow it out through your open mouth. Continue for several breaths, drawing the air in through your feet and up through your body and then blowing it out slowly and calmly.

"Imagine that as you draw the air up through your body, you are sweeping all of the contracted energy — blocks, hesitations, illnesses, weaknesses, and fears that keep you from being your highest, best self — along with it. Breathe up through your feet and your body, sweeping along all contracted energies and then blowing them out with the air calmly and slowly. Feel the movement of air and the sweeping of energy as vividly as you can.

"Now imagine that as the swept-up energy hits the open air, it bursts into a shower of colorful sparks. The bright sparks sprinkle down light and positive healing energy throughout your body."

Breath Awareness

"Gently close your eyes, breathing in and out through your mouth with the jaw hanging loosely open. You're breathing slowly, quietly, calmly, gently. Feel your belly moving with each breath, expanding gently with each inhale, drawing in life, and releasing gently. With each exhale, let life go. Every inhale, fill your belly. Every exhale, let go . . .

"Now allow yourself to breathe in and out through your nose and mouth at the same time so that exactly the same amount of air is passing in and out through both openings while continuing to take each breath from deep in your belly.

"Continue this breathing for the next few minutes with equal amounts of air passing through your nose and mouth, your belly gently rising and falling with each easy breath as your eyes remain softly closed.

"Stay with your breath. Focus on it moving down into your body and then release it up through your body. Continue to release the tension in your jaw, then your neck, and finally your shoulders."

Daily Health Reminders

1. Follow your nutritionist's or medical doctor's recommendations for eating. This may include eating soft foods only or eliminating sodium and/or fatty foods in your diet.

2. Drink plenty of water (e.g., six to eight glasses a day). If you are on a thickened consistency diet, thicken liquids as shown by your speech-language pathologist. If you are unable to meet your hydration needs, make sure to notify your physician. Dehydration can cause tiredness, a decrease in mental acuity, mood swings, and damage to your vital organs.

3. Avoid excessive use of sugar and caffeine unless stated otherwise by your nutritionist or medical doctor.

4. Avoid smoking and secondhand smoke inhalation. They both cause dehydration and have been found to cause cancer.

5. Exercise 30 minutes every day. If needed, break the exercises up into five-minute stretches or small walks. If in a wheelchair, stretch your arms and neck. Massage your hands and face. Follow through on any exercises given to you by your therapists.

6. Spend at least 30 minutes every day doing something fun. Take a break. Do something creative or simply breathe and clear your mind of what has collected throughout the day.

7. Be positive and surround yourself with positive, affirming people.

Chapter 2: Communication

It is important to build rapport and self-esteem with the client so he is motivated in therapy. The client may be worried about many things such as:

- loss of physical abilities
- loss of independence
- high medical expenses
- loss of control

All of these can contribute to depression and anger in the client as well as in the primary caregivers. Acknowledging the client's emotions and maintaining a positive and productive relationship is a primary goal in therapy. The following techniques can be tried with clients to develop good, open communication.

The Disarming Technique

Find some truth in what the client is saying, even if you feel it's incorrect. Acceptance is not agreement. For example, the client might say, "You don't know the first thing about my condition. You're a lousy therapist." A good response is, "It's true I don't have **your** insight into your condition, but through my education and work with many clients who have similar conditions, I have gained some insight and understanding. Please help me learn more." When you use this type of disarming response, you're showing the client that you're acknowledging his feelings.

Empathy

By paraphrasing what the client is saying or feeling, you are acknowledging what he is going through and showing concern. Being empathetic will show the client that you understand what he is thinking and feeling. You'll validate the client's feelings which will ultimately lead to greater bonding. For example, if a client says, "I can't take it any more. I've had it." You might say, "I hear you. You're frustrated and feel that you've gone through so much already."

Inquiry

Probe for more information by asking what the client is thinking or feeling. Look beyond negative comments, moodiness, or apathy to the client's true concerns by asking sensitive and thoughtful questions. For example, you might say, "You don't seem very interested in your exercises today. Is something bothering you?" or "I sense something is on your mind today."

Chapter 2, *continued*

Positive Reinforcement

Make genuinely positive comments to clients even when you're not happy with how things are going. If you notice something positive, mention it. For example, "Good eye contact, you're so alert today," or "I see you're really trying." You want to say something positive even when a client is not making significant progress.

While helping clients with their exercises, remember to always explain what you're doing. Use positive statements to keep clients alert, on target, and motivated. After completing an exercise, say things like, "Good, great, that's it, good try," or "It's nice to spend time with you." Be sincere.

Avoid negative statements. Don't say, "No, do the exercise this way." Instead you might say, "Good try! Let's do it again this way."

Be short and to the point. Instead of saying, "Okay now Mr. Harrison, I'd like you to pick up your left hand." You could say, "Please raise your left hand. That's good." Short commands with an acknowledgement that the exercise was performed correctly are appropriate and efficient.

Things to Consider When Communicating

- If a client's speech becomes unintelligible or difficult to understand, try saying, "Sometimes it's difficult for me to understand what you're saying. Try saying one word at a time. Take a new breath before each word. Say each word loudly." If the client doesn't seem to understand you, say each statement individually with adequate time for response. You might also ask the client to open his mouth and jaw wider during word formation.

- Hearing loss might inhibit your client's communication. If so, the client will benefit from your increased eye contact by naturally reading your lips. An audiological examination is indicated if hearing loss is suspected.

Chapter 2, continued

- When giving directions or conversing:

  - Make sure the client can see your face.

  - Maintain eye contact.

  - Initially state your name and occupation.

  - Use short sentences that explain what you're going to do therapeutically. "We're going to work with your lips today . . ." Wait for the client to process the information and then continue with, " . . . to try to help stop your drooling."

- Explain every detail of the therapy session, including rationale with the family, caregivers, nurses, doctor, and other therapists. The more involved these people are, the better for the client's progress.

  Remember to include the client in any conversations you have. Talk to him even if there is no eye contact, gestures, or verbal response. Try to establish a system of yes/no responses with arm squeeze or eye gaze.

- Due to the number of therapies the client is involved in, it will be necessary to create a routine time schedule. Discuss with the client and caregivers which times are best for therapeutic intervention involving exercises. Remember that factors such as time of medication and feeding may interfere with the client's attentive state.

  It's important to be flexible when setting up the program because each client is different. Adjust the therapy program to the client's specific needs. As exercises are added into the program, you may wish to delete previous exercises to shorten or maintain the time schedule.

- If the client's voice becomes inaudible or his writing becomes illegible, a picture or written communication board can be useful. The client can point to the desired picture, word, or sentence. An eye gaze method is often effective for patients with severe tremors because they can scan from a field of many choices provided visually.

  Commercial communication boards with voice capabilities are also available. There are a variety of models on the market for purchase or rental. When using a communication board, give the client plenty of time to locate the picture, word, or sentence. It's helpful to practice with various types of communication boards before any purchase or rental to determine which one is most effective.

- It's common for affected individuals to experience changes in vision. Loss in peripheral vision or visual neglect are commonly associated with a stroke. Consult an ophthalmologist for the type and scope of the client's visual disturbance.

Emotional Associations with the Body Segments

When someone has a physical problem such as tension in the neck, it can create emotional problems. The person might repress his feelings and/or have difficulty expressing himself. It can also go the other way in that when someone has emotional problems, the problems might manifest themselves physically. For example, if someone is repressing his emotions, he might have neck tension or pain in his chest. Helping this person learn how to express his emotions can lead to physical improvement.

Body Segment	Emotional Association
ocular (eye) and oral area	difficulty expressing feelings shows difficulty in rational thinking
neck area	division between rational thoughts and actual feelings chokes down feelings difficulty expressing feelings
shoulder area	doesn't take responsibility or takes on too much responsibility judgment (including self-judgment)
chest area	restricts the flow of emotions heartache or heartbreak
diaphragm and abdominal area	lack of emotional and intrapersonal power fear of losing oneself to one's feelings
pelvic area	difficulty talking about sex and elimination fear of our primary survival needs or of losing control to our primal self

(Teeguarden)

Projecting the Positive

Positive messages start any session off on better footing. They can counteract negative messages going on in the individual's mind that may have been there since childhood or appeared as a result of a recent decline in function. Negative messages can provoke pessimism. Help your client learn to assert the positive with the examples on the following pages.

Chapter 2, continued

Negative Statements	Positive Affirmations
I'll have to . . .	It's in my best interest to . . .
I'd hate to see you fail.	I want to see you succeed.
We can't fight this.	We can improve this by . . .
This creates a problem.	This opens up an opportunity.
You're no good at that.	You're improving at that.
This is impossible.	This requires special effort.
I've just been here three months, but . . .	I've observed carefully and . . .
You just don't understand.	I haven't made it clear.
I was wondering if you could . . .	When will you be able . . .
Here's why we failed . . .	Here's what we learned.
If only you had . . .	Next time . . .
Here's what you have to do . . .	Here's what we can do.
I disagree with you.	I understand you would like to consider . . .
My life is finished.	My life is different and well worth living.
I can't and won't deal with this.	I am doing the best I know how. Do you have any suggestions on how I can deal with it more effectively? I am open to suggestions.
I am just getting worse and worse.	I am handling whatever happens.
Why does everything happen to me?	Difficulties happen to everyone. I am sure others have also gone through this. Is there someone I can talk to who has gone through this and can offer advice and solace?
This is unbearable.	I can adjust and live through this.
I will never be able to do any of the things that are important to me.	I will get to do many of the things that I enjoy doing.

Chapter 2, continued

More Positive Comments for Clients

Repeat these during the session for support, copy them on daily homework sheets, and/or post them in the room for motivation.

Act as though it is impossible to fail.

We are not retreating; we are just advancing in another direction.

Everything is for the good.

Pain is blocked energy. Let it pass through you with each breath exhalation.

Find the space between two thoughts. Put your thoughts into boxes to take a break. Breathe in the middle. Your thoughts will be waiting for you when you are ready.

I would like you to suspend doubt for the next two days so creativity and learning can flourish.

The word courage in French means from the heart. It takes great heart to care, to be vulnerable, and to train your body and mind again. I respect you for your continued effort.

Chapter 3:
Posture and Stretches

> Consult the client's physician before beginning any stretching or exercise program.

Posture

Help the client recognize the benefits of a daily stretch and tone program by explaining how improper posture affects respiration and rhythm of speech. By correcting improper posture, the client's vocal quality can be improved.

Improper posture is characterized by:

- head and neck extended forward
- sunken chest
- rounded shoulders
- leaning to one side
- protruding abdomen
- slouched lower back with no lumbar support
- knees extending beyond support of seat

Secondary effects of improper posture include:

- low voice level
- breathy voice
- higher risk for aspiration
- coughing
- food spillage
- overall fatigue
- improper eye contact
- poor hand-eye coordination

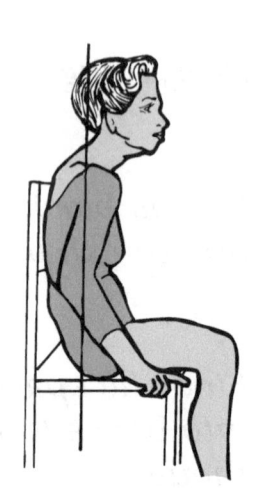

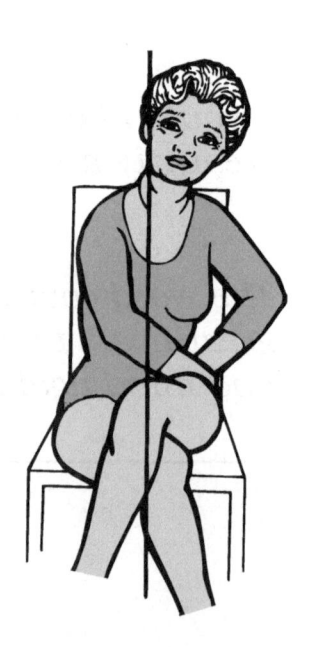

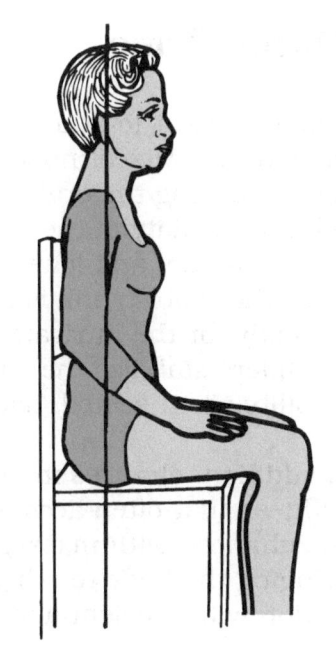

Chapter 3, *continued*

To correct improper posture, begin by having the client sit down. Proper posture can be visually identified by drawing an imaginary line down the client's body with equal alignment on either side. The shoulders and buttocks are back and the legs are fully supported by the bottom of the seat. The line check for posture can be assessed from the side and front, showing equal body distribution on either side of the line.

Posture has a direct link to fatigue due to an interference with adequate respiration. Changes in posture will allow for deeper respiration which will create a louder voice. By changing posture, muscle tone is improved. This, along with increasing caloric and nutritional food intake, can give a client energy to improve voicing, speech skills, and gross and fine motor movement. When a client is tired, she isn't able to function to the best of her ability.

If a client is exhibiting shallow breathing due to improper posture, she'll have an insufficient air supply for voicing. The client will only be able to produce one or two words in a weak, nearly inaudible voice and then mouth the remaining words.

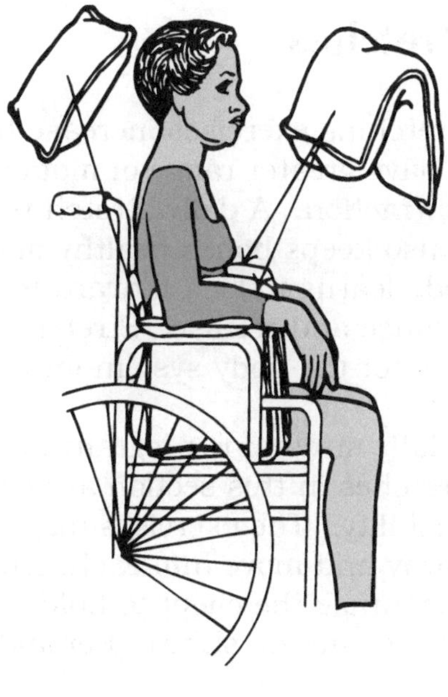

Teach the client to sit up properly using pillows or supports under her arms and behind her lower back.

It's important that the client change positions frequently throughout the day. This will help the client rest her musculature, stretch her back, and relieve tension in her neck. Having clients sit too long in one position can increase drooling as well as weaken and misalign neck musculature.

The general rule is to keep a client seated for no more than one hour at a time. If the client is able to walk, taking a walk and doing some basic calisthenics are recommended. Keep in mind that the best exercise for good posture is to use good posture. Daily body stretches and exercises are listed on the following pages.

> To make a low back support, fold a small towel in half and roll it into a cylindrical shape. Place the rolled-up towel between the client's lower back and the back of the chair. This will maintain the arch of the client's lower back.

The Oral-Facial Therapy Exercise Book
2021 Edition

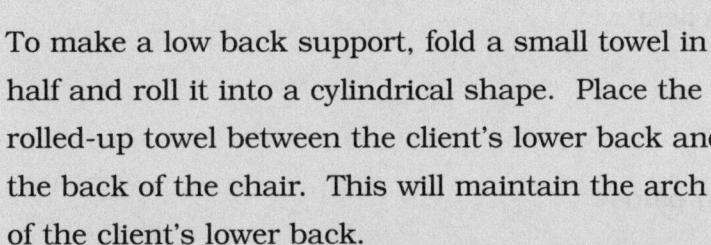

Muscle Tone

It is important to address atypical muscle tone and movement patterns prior to working on the mouth. Mixed muscle tone throughout the body can lead to fluctuations in muscle control during the oral-motor movements needed for speech and swallowing. Therefore, to achieve mobility of the oral-motor mechanism, shoulder and trunk stability is necessary. The shoulders and lower body work as an anchor to support the movements of the face. Once the lower trunk is stabilized, you can pursue the finer points of stability throughout the body for the intricate movements needed for precise oral-motor range of motion (e.g., shoulders stabilize the jaw, jaw stabilizes the tongue). To help the client achieve trunk stability when seated, use pillows and/or a tray for support.

In addition, changes in posture can help reduce inappropriate spasming as well as the stiffness that often accompanies weakened low tone areas. Overall body balance can also be enhanced with massage, acupressure, and stretching and strengthening exercises. Bringing the body to a higher level of postural stability can give the oral cavity freedom of motion with efficient and precise functional movement.

Stretches

Stretching exercises increase the ability of the tissues to lengthen. This enables joints to have greater range of motion before meeting resistance from tension and muscle contraction. A daily stretch routine keeps the muscles toned and flexible, reducing atrophy. It also keeps bones healthy and strong. Stretching is a series of regular movements that the body learns to look forward to. Stretching exercises can also provide emotional and physical balance and release. Stretching opens the breath, allowing new energy and vital force to enter the body system for concentration, vocal output, and renewed confidence.

A daily stretching program will give the client energy rather than exhaust her. The body stretches in this section are for the client to perform between meals to maintain tone and flexibility. The exercises may be performed one at a time or collectively. Have the client go slowly and move into each new position gently. Avoid abrupt or sudden movements. Encourage the client to hold each stretch for at least a 10-second count or as long as stated without undue strain. Remind the client to move slowly out of position.

The degree of stretch or the range of motion may increase over a period of time. The best results are achieved when the exercises are performed one to three times daily. Simple stretches will help the client:

- maintain posture
- relieve aches and pains
- feel rejuvenated

Chapter 3, *continued*

○ stimulate appetite

○ strengthen and tone musculature

The stretches will strengthen arm, shoulder, and neck musculature. Arm stretches and exercises can be performed from a standing or seated position. These exercises are excellent additions to therapy programs for clients with:

- vocal strain
- temporomandibular joint problems
- reduced range of motion for the neck
- poor posture
- laryngectomy with radical neck dissection

If a physical limitation such as unilateral weakness or paralysis limits full body stretching, the client may choose to work her unaffected side or limbs only. However, it is important to try to work bilaterally. A referral to a physical therapist and/or occupational therapist to establish a client's physical capability will help you develop a plan of stretching, toning, and range of motion.

Remind the client that stretching is meant to feel good. Provide a simple model or help the client adjust her body into position. Have her move her limbs gently and freely without force. Remind the client to only move to the point of a comfortable stretch. It is wise to have the client stretch up to the point of pain and then just let the stretch relax. The goal is for relaxation and expansion, not for tension or fear of stretching. Remind the client to take deep full breaths as she stretches. She will start to see improvement in flexibility, strength, pain reduction, and freedom of movement.

The Stretch Routine

Start with the first exercise and do a routine or you can start anywhere. It is better to do at least one exercise versus none.

- Rise and Shine Stimulating Breath Exercise
- Full-Face Scrunch
- Hand Crawl
- Upper Body Stretching Exercises
- Lower Body Stretching Exercises

Hand Crawl

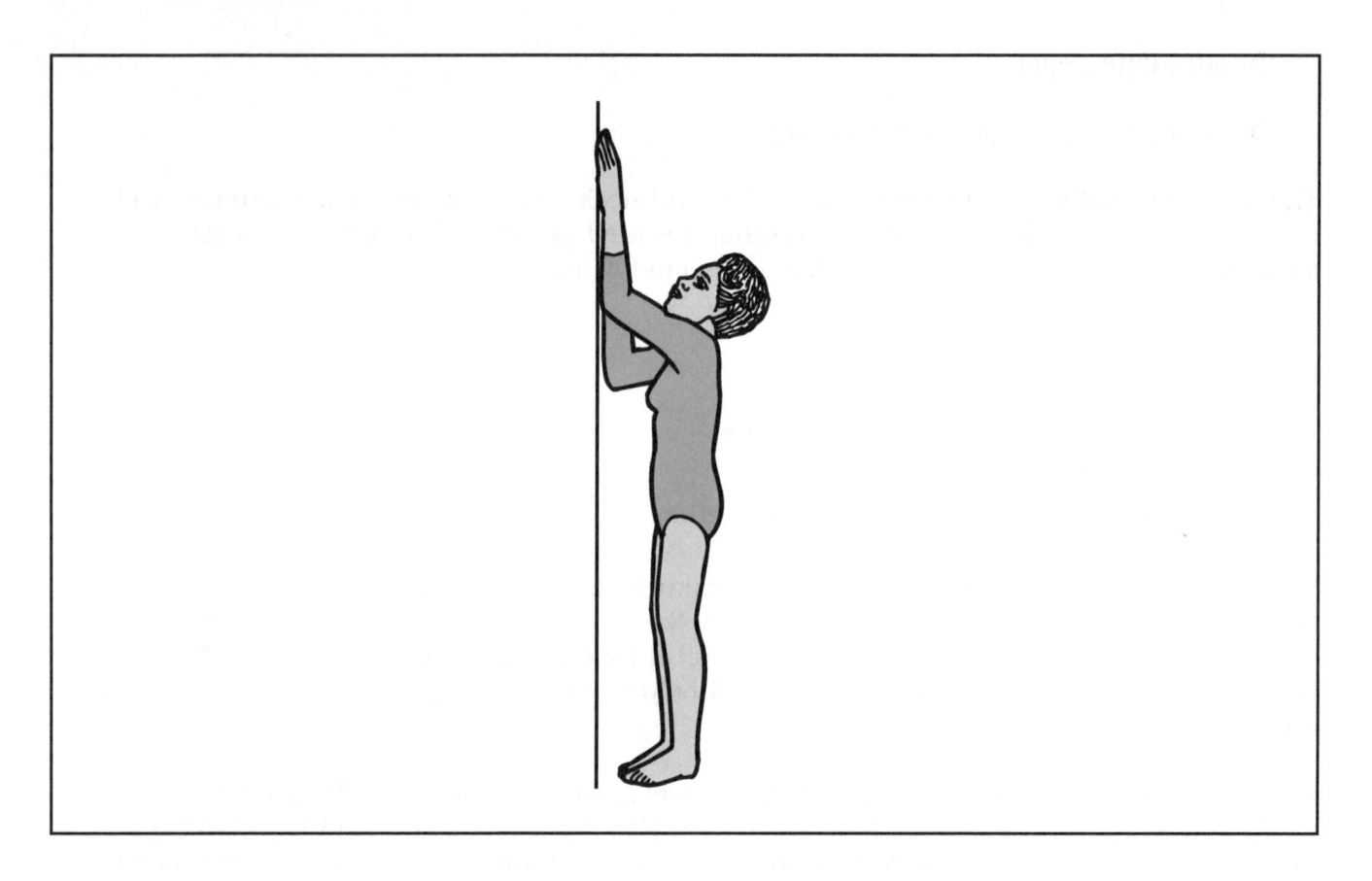

Chapter 3, continued

Stand facing a wall and put your hands on the wall at stomach level. Crawl them little by little up the wall, alternating left and right hands. Stop at a predetermined point or until you can't stretch any further. Then slowly crawl hands back down the wall to stomach level.

> Note: This exercise is particularly beneficial for clients with laryngectomies involving radical neck dissections.

Benefit

- strengthens head, neck, and arm musculature

Chapter 3, *continued*

Upper Body Stretching Exercises

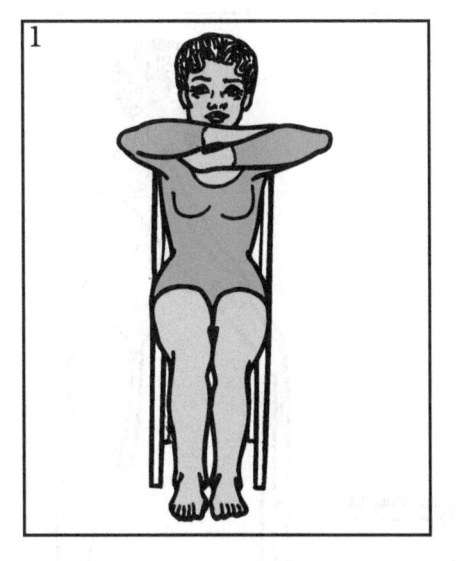

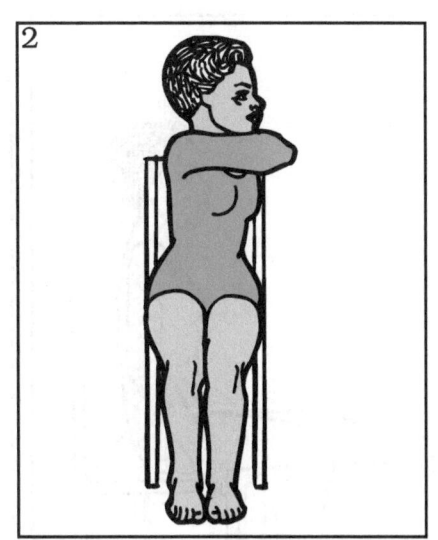

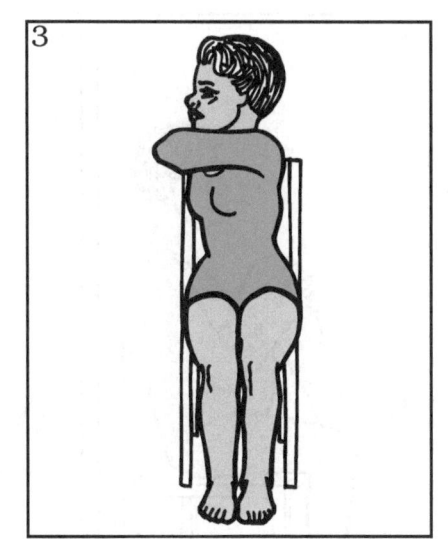

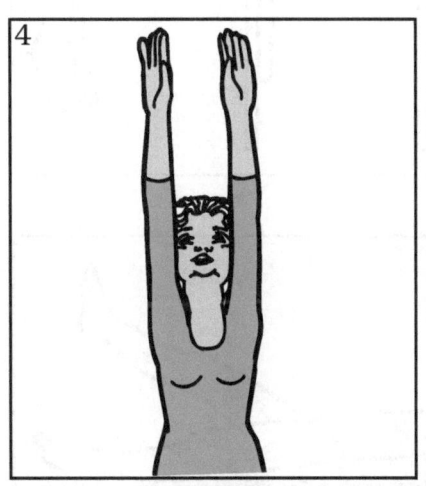

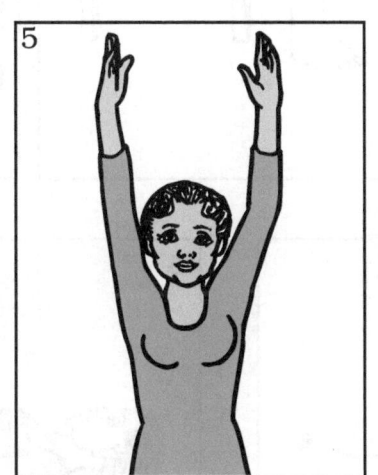

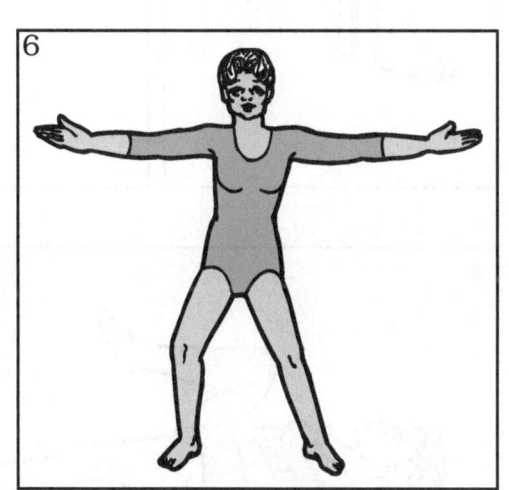

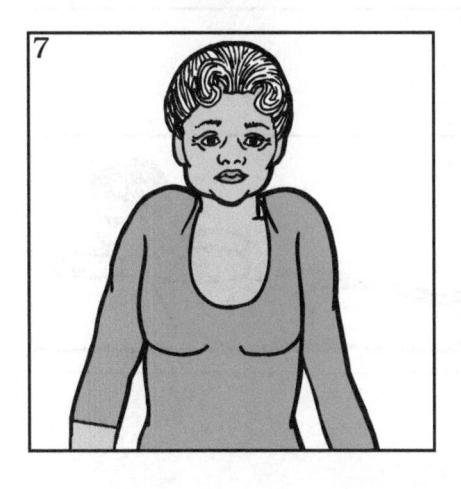

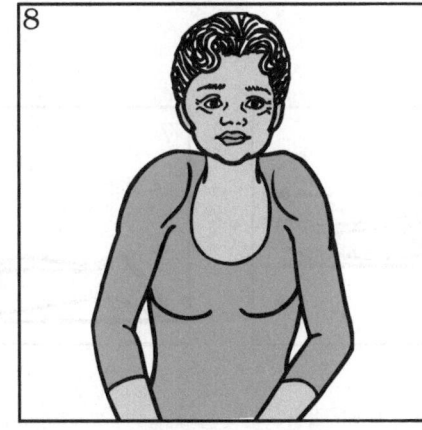

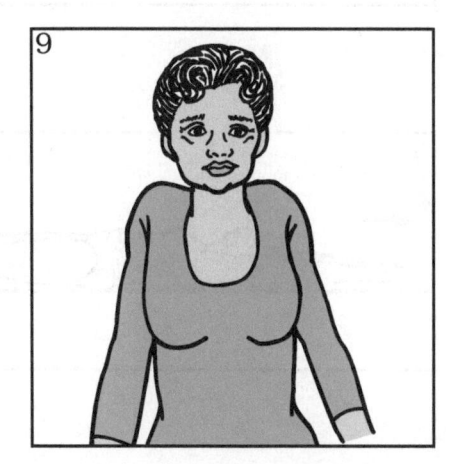

The Oral-Facial Therapy Exercise Book
2021 Edition

Copyright © 2021

Lower Body Stretching Exercises

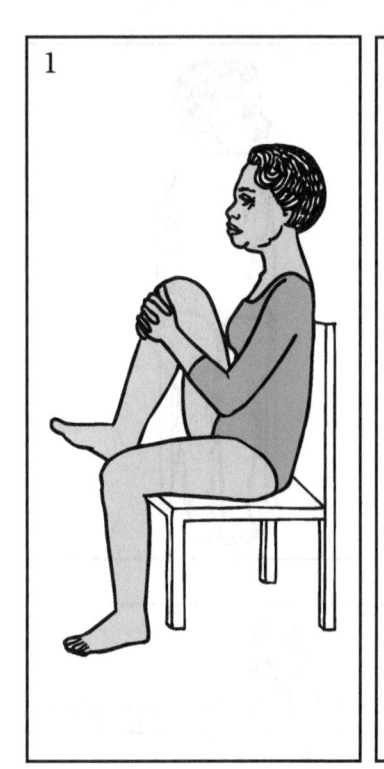

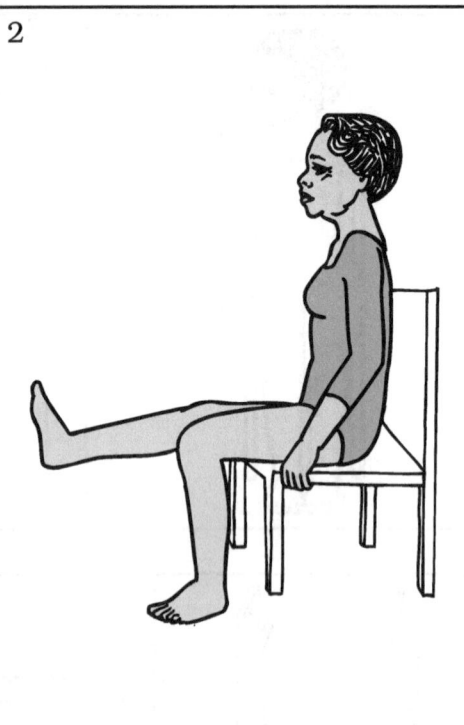

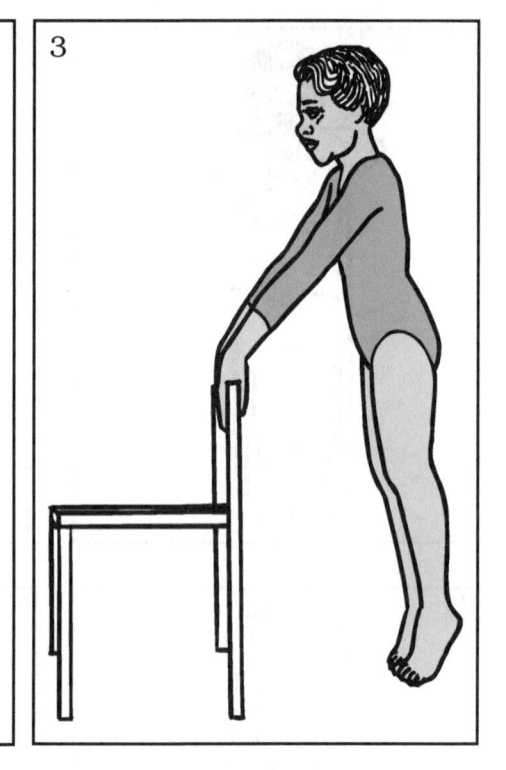

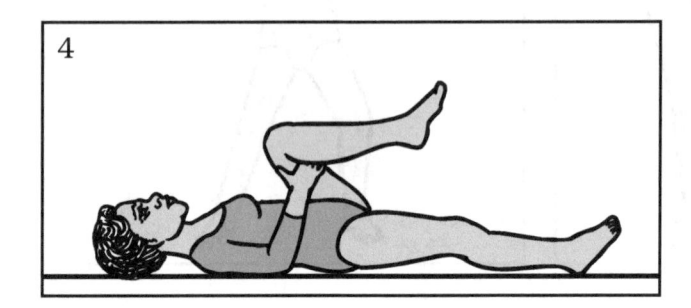

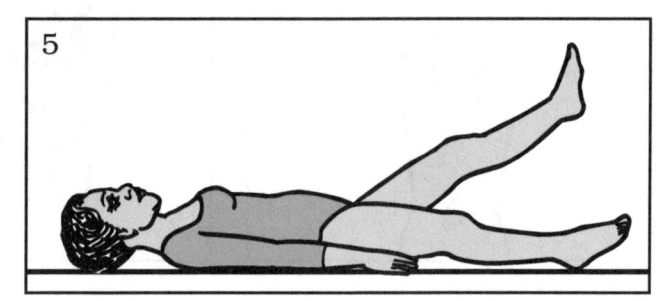

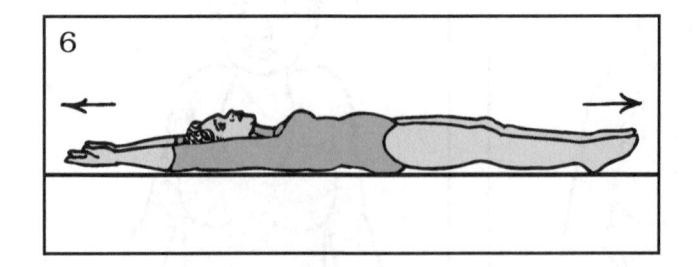

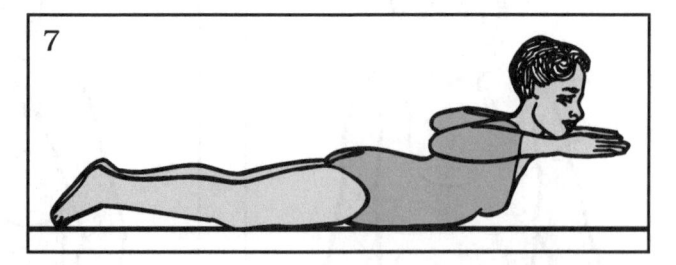

Chapter 3, *continued*

The Oral-Facial Therapy Exercise Book
2021 Edition

Chapter 4:
Drooling Management

Drooling affects the general well-being of an individual and may present daily problems for the caregiver. The goals of drooling management are to promote a better quality of life for speech, swallowing, and social interactions.

Basically, saliva aids in protecting the teeth from decay and the gums from inflammation and periodontal disease. Saliva keeps the oral mucosa comfortably moist, acts as a lubricant for swallowing, and works as a solvent for facilitating taste. Saliva is anti-bacterial and helps reduce breath odor by cleaning the mouth. Average production of saliva is between .5 to 1.5 liters daily in adults. This diminishes with age, depending on environmental stimuli and conditions. Saliva also promotes the breakdown of carbohydrates and proteins.

	Drooling Level Indicator
Mild Drooling	can be distinguished as spill of saliva onto the lips but not beyond the lip border
Moderate Drooling	saliva reaches the chin
Severe Drooling	saliva drips onto clothing
Profuse Drooling	saliva spills onto everything (e.g., books and equipment)
Anterior Spill	visible anterior oral or labial (lip) which can create impaired oral-motor function affecting speech, swallowing, and breathing
Posterior Spill	oral secretions that pool or collect in the back of the throat (hypopharynx) where, in normal situations, they should stimulate a swallowing reflex. Posterior spills will cause retention sublingually, in buccal pools, in the pharynx, and in the faucial isthmus. This posterior pooling of liquid and the absence of a normal swallow creates coughing, gagging, congested breathing, bad breath, and vomiting which can lead to aspiration into the trachea.

The causes of posterior drooling can be related to severe oral-motor dysfunction, pharyngeal sensory deficit, and/or a central disruption of the sensorimotor connection which interferes with the swallowing reflex.

Weakened or paralyzed musculature combined with a sagging and inappropriate habitual head-down posture increases the flow of saliva as well as the amount of liquids and foods coming out of the mouth. This, in turn, will cause drooling. Treatments to improve body positioning and posture along with oral-motor interventions are integral in the management

Chapter 4, continued

of drooling. You might want to contact a physical therapist or occupational therapist for input on exercises; transferring techniques; assistive equipment available for improved head control; balanced muscle tone; and/or jaw, shoulder, and lower body stabilization.

It is best to work toward appropriate jaw tone and stability, lip closure, improved swallowing competency, and sensory discrimination. Remember that practice makes permanent, but not necessarily perfect. A reduction in overall drooling through many of the techniques listed will help the individual to better adapt and acclimate to his body's physical limitations. Elimination of drooling is the goal but any help that can be attained to limit and manage drooling must also be seen as success and documented as such. Use the Drooling Level Indicator to chart progress.

Interventions for Drooling

Posture/Positioning	See information for posture and positioning in Chapter 3.
Oral-motor Interventions	See sensory stimulation, massage to lips and cheeks, intra-oral massage, lip exercises, facial massage, neck releases and stretches, and jaw interventions throughout the book.
Chin Cups	Chin cups can be used to collect the saliva. However, combined interventions (e.g., improved posture, facial massage) show greater success than solely using the cup to reduce spillage to the chin, face, and clothing.
Auditory Cues	Auditory cues are used to remind the individual to swallow at regular intervals. These cues could be someone saying "swallow" or a bell or a beeper that goes off every minute or two to remind the person to swallow.

Chapter 4, continued

Behavior Modification Behavior modification is intended to break habits, bring awareness to the spillage of liquids, give praise to appropriate saliva management, and to build self-esteem needed for continued instruction. "Suck and Swallow" is a valuable prompt that can be given verbally, written on a card for a visual reminder, or played on a tape player. Using the chin cup to show how much saliva has been collected will informally gauge how much the individual has been listening or remembering to use the cue.

The goal is to be able to decrease the cues, the behavior modification intervention, and the direct therapy managed care of the individual's saliva spillage problem.

Other Tips for Managing the Effects of Drooling

- Use a plastic-backed absorbent pad (e.g., Chux) as a bib to absorb the excessive spillage onto the chest and pants. This pad can also be placed on a pillow to absorb liquid during rest time.

- Plastic shields and/or soft plastic coverings are effective in protecting books and equipment.

- Protect the skin from constant wet rash with topical creams. Topical cream is frequently used around ostomy sites to avoid infection and rash. Contact the client's primary physician or a dermatologist for further information.

Find the Saliva Case Management Information Form in the Appendix.

Chapter 5: Stimulation Therapy

Stimulation treatments are designed to improve the client's cognitive and motor abilities in the case of head trauma, cerebral palsy, low-functioning developmental delay, stroke with cognitive impairments, or Alzheimer's disease. The activities described can integrate naturally into family visitation and therapy sessions. These stimulation techniques are important for all caregivers to do to help alert and orient the client as much as possible. The therapy should:

- occur three to five times per day
- be in 10 – 20 minute sessions
- use a variety of techniques
- not be painful or noxious

It's important to document all stimulation techniques used in order to evaluate the effectiveness of intervention. You might use the Stimulation Chart on page 62 to report:

- baseline responses
- pretreatment status
- target stimulation applied
- client responses
- observations

Examples of Stimulation (See Materials List on page 13.)

1. Auditory Stimulation

Music, everyday sounds, and speech can alert and orient the client.

○ Music

- favorite songs
- musical instruments like drums, whistles, noisemakers, harmonicas, bells, buzzers (present in loud/soft and long/staccato contrasts)
- music therapy by a registered music therapist

○ Environmental

- home/outdoor sounds – dog barking, door slamming, teapot whistling, programming microwave, television playing, toilet flushing, phone ringing, birds chirping, police car siren
- speech – family, friends, co-workers, talk shows, favorite movies

Chapter 5, *continued*

2. Tactile Stimulation

Check the client's chart for any allergic sensitivities and/or allergies prior to use in therapy. You might also question the family, caregivers, nursing staff, or dietitian.

- human touch – holding; slowly stroking arms, face, and hair; massaging; grasping palm; tickling; lightly stroking with fingertips; brushing hair; lightly brushing skin on arms, legs, or cheeks with a soft bristle painter's brush

- textures – feather, sandpaper, dry washcloth, wet washcloth, cotton swab, tongue blade, flowers, leaves, grass, brush, comb, fur, foam, or any other type of soft, hard, bumpy, smooth, or coarse texture

- temperature – ice-cold washcloth, warm washcloth, neutral temperature items like Play–doh or a textured ball

Verbally and visually introduce the object/texture to your client, even if you're unsure as to whether the client is comprehending the message.

Depending on the client's functioning level, orient him to facial body parts, to his location, his name, the time of day, your name, his occupation, and/or his relation to you. Ask for basic responses like eye twitch, eye open, or mouth open.

- Begin with the client's palms.

- Progress to the underside of the arms, then the neck.

- Continue onto the cheeks.

- Avoid direct contact with eyes and nose areas.

3. Olfactory Stimulation

- strong familiar smells – perfume, aftershave, food odors (coffee, vanilla, garlic), cedar, rubber

Avoid toxic items, medicines, detergents, alcohol, ammonia, or any other chemical which could cause a reaction (e.g., skin or eye irritation and burning).

Introduce each item visually and verbally before a 5 to 10 second olfactory stimulation. Hold the item at least 12 inches out and below the client's face. Describe common uses for each item and familiar places the odor may be detected. Encourage clients to identify the odor with cues if necessary.

Chapter 5, *continued*

4. Gustatory Stimulation (Taste)

Check the client's chart for any allergic sensitivities or allergies and/or any dietary restrictions prior to use in therapy. You might also question the family, caregivers, nursing staff, or dietitian.

Exercise caution with individuals exhibiting any swallowing difficulties. Taste stimulation is not advised with individuals who are receiving nothing by mouth (NPO). A swallowing therapist (SLP skilled in swallowing therapy) can recommend consistencies which can be tolerated safely.

- favorite and familiar tastes – any comfort food or nonalcoholic beverage the individual enjoys such as spaghetti, pie, sauce, jelly, or chocolate

- taste contrast – salty/bitter, sweet/sour, mildly spicy/bland

Increasing taste awareness may allow the individual to increase tolerance to oral-motor stimulation and to increase appetite for oral feedings. Wrap the food item in cheesecloth or organza for the individual to suck on. Thicken any liquids to manage transition time through the oral and pharyngeal cavity. When using taste stimulation, keep in mind that sweet receptors are found on the front of the tongue, and salty and sour taste receptors are found a bit farther back and to the sides. Bitter taste receptors are positioned toward the back of the tongue. Various types of food items for taste stimulation are:

- Popsicles
- fruit smoothies
- fruit puree
- vegetable puree
- Mrs. Dash's
- cinnamon
- vanilla
- jams
- jellies
- syrup

Present these items chilled, frozen, at room temperature, or slightly warmed as is tolerated and deemed safe for oral feeding.

The client might also benefit from:

- thermal stimulation (iced stimulation designed to trigger an immediate swallow reflex)
- intra-oral massage (digital or swab massage in the intra-oral cavity)
- toning (stretching, elongating, and firming musculature)
- range of motion exercises
- passive exercises (performed by the client or aide without assistance from target musculature)
- active exercises (client actively attempts to move target musculature)

The Oral-Facial Therapy Exercise Book
2021 Edition

Chapter 5, *continued*

5. Visual Stimulation

Any of the following items can be presented to the client to increase awareness, cognition, attention, naming, memory, and orientation.

- familiar photos, videos, movies, objects, toys, tools, food, functional daily items (e.g., pen, comb, purse, mirror, toothbrush)

- variation of lighting – sunlight, room light on or off, penlight or flashlight in darkened room (give light to client to manipulate and track)

- variation of color – bright or contrasting clothing or objects

6. Vestibular (Movement) Stimulation

Movement helps increase body awareness as well as increase vocalization and communication. The client needs to be upright, alert, and have relatively good head support and trunk stability in order to eat and communicate well.

- changes in positioning – transfers to and from bed, therapy apparatus, water therapy, occupational and physical therapy

7. Intra-oral Stimulation

Note: Remember to wear gloves when working in and around a client's mouth.

The following stimulation activities and all other passive exercises may be introduced at all levels of cognition and at all ages. For the client who is orally hypersensitive, stimulation to the oral cavity will reduce tactile discomfort to textured foods. It will also decrease an excessive gag reflex. For the client who is orally hyposensitive, this stimulation will increase oral sensitivity and muscle activity thereby improving feeding, articulation, and resonance.

Use a toothette, gauze, and/or soft bristle toothbrush to brush the client's inner cheek walls. If using a toothette, twirl the stick in your hand to provide a circular stimulation to the inner cheeks. From your client's cheeks, move down to the lower gums, stimulating the outer gum surface with a soft brushing motion or use your index finger to apply firm pressure, gliding front to back and back to front once. Gradually increase tolerance to five times up and back.

Take the toothette and begin at the alveolar ridge. Brush or twirl it backward along the hard palate. Gradually increase stimulation to the soft palate as tolerated. Once the client can tolerate toothette stimulation to the soft palate, twirl the toothette over to the left gum line and move it back to midline. Repeat to right gum line. Stop short of the gag reflex.

Chapter 5, continued

Facial Sensory Stimulation Exercises

Introduce the following exercises as passive exercises for clients who are unable to follow commands and show no response, but would benefit from sensory stimulation. The exercises also reduce further atrophy and stimulate muscle activity.

1. **Brush Cheeks**
    Use a soft bristle, two-inch wide paintbrush and make rapid upward motions on the client's cheeks.

2. **Circular Cheek Pinch**
    Gently pinch the client's cheek musculature with your index finger and thumb, beginning at the lip corners, moving up to the cheekbone, and then circling down and back to the masseter muscle. Continue the circular motion or randomly pinch the cheek musculature.

3. **Ice Cube Stimulation to Cheeks**
    Apply an ice cube to the one of the client's cheeks by stroking backward from lip corner toward the ear lobe. With each stroke, start at the lip corner again, and fan back and upward, stopping at the cheekbone. Do not allow the ice cube to touch the client's eyes, ears, and/or nose. After each stroke, wipe the cheek dry using an upward motion. Discontinue if client strongly objects or shows aversive reaction. Do not overstimulate.

4. **Cheek Tap**
    Tap cheeks and temporomandibular joint in a rhythmic fashion. Tap both sides simultaneously. This increases jaw stability and cheek tone.

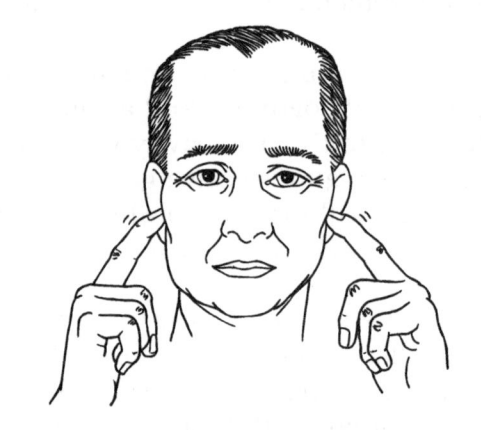

The Oral-Facial Therapy Exercise Book
2021 Edition

Washcloth Stimulation

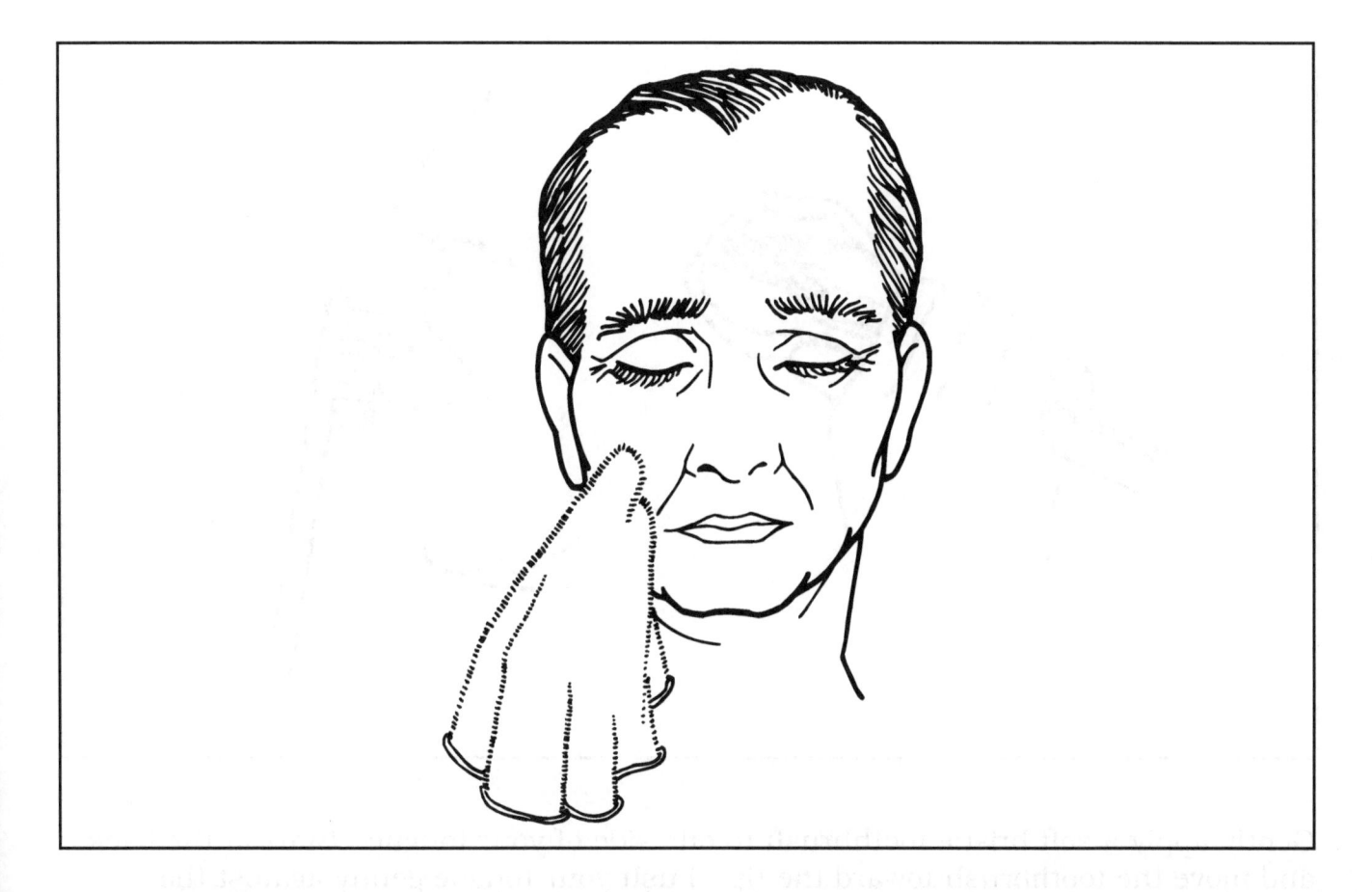

Chapter 5, *continued*

Go around the entire face in a large sweeping massage. Then pat the entire face in a tapping motion.

Gently squeeze a small portion of skin between your index finger and thumb with washcloth. Release quickly. Continue this around the entire face.

Switch from dry to wet washcloth, varying from cool to warm every couple of minutes for a change in stimulation. Avoid eyes and nostril openings. Perform no longer than 10 minutes.

Benefits

- stretches cheek musculature
- improves facial tone
- assists in orientation

Toothbrush Stimulation

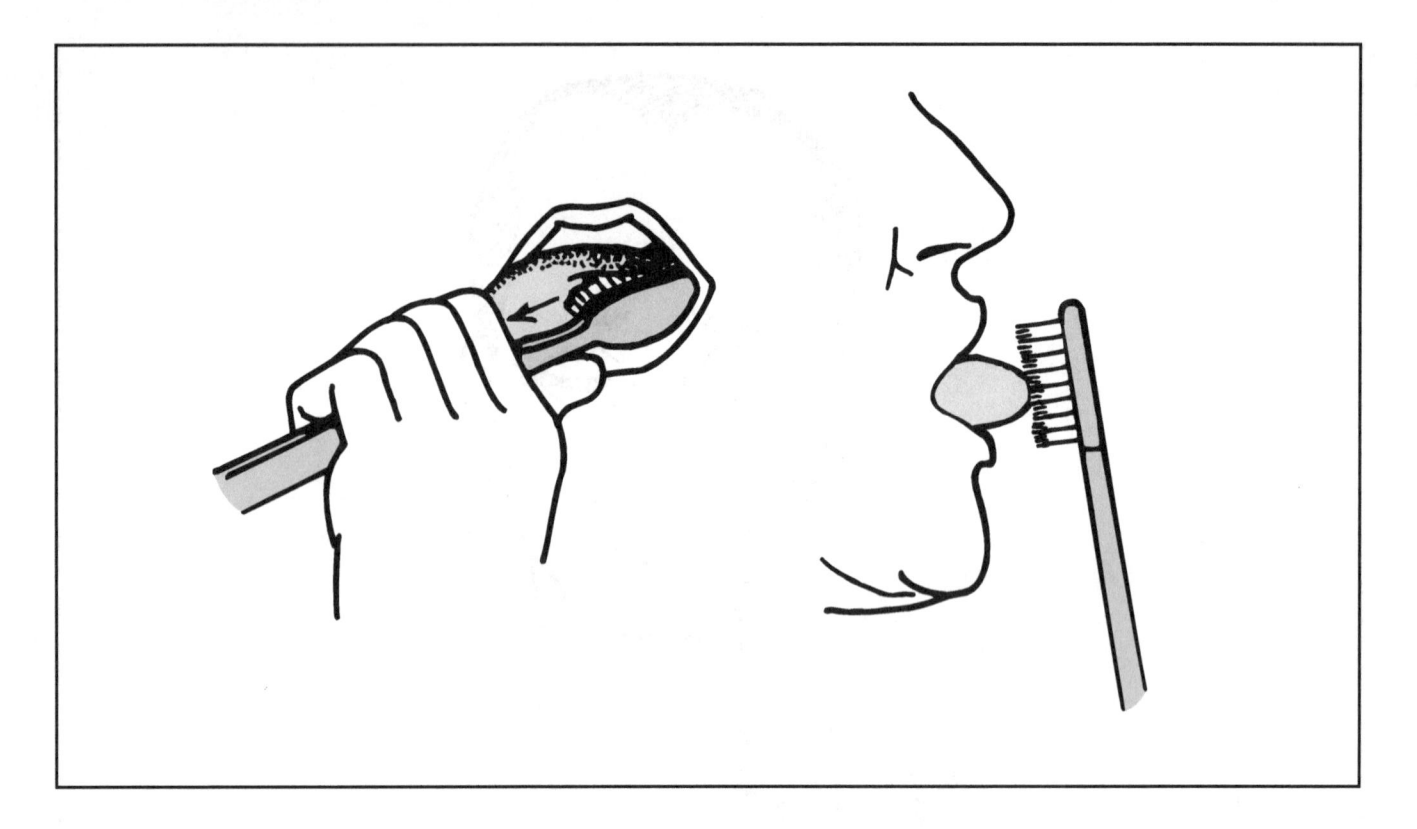

Chapter 5, continued

Gently apply a soft bristle toothbrush to one side of your tongue. Start in the back and move the toothbrush toward the tip. Push your tongue gently against the toothbrush. Do the same thing on the other side. Repeat once.

Then brush the tip of your tongue up with toothbrush. Incorporate this exercise into regular toothbrushing activity.

This exercise can also be done with a fingertip, toothette, or iced cotton-tip applicator.

Benefits

- stimulates lateral widening of tongue
- increases range of motion laterally
- promotes tongue tip awareness

Note: This exercise can be done by the therapist or caregiver if the client is unable to perform or when teaching the client how to perform.

Chapter 5, continued

Intervention Tools

1. Microphone

The use of a microphone to amplify speech is effective in oral-motor training. Many individuals will try harder to articulate more precisely when the sound is amplified because the feedback loop for correction is emphasized.

2. Music

Individuals with Down syndrome, dementia, Parkinson's disease, dysarthria, stroke, or any unspecified neurological impairment may have experienced failure after failure trying to produce intelligible speech. Music has been found to help these people communicate. Music bypasses the left side of the brain and goes right to where music is processed. Many times the individual can learn new songs with new words. Being able to say a few words, even with delayed response time, gives the individual a sense of control and coordination. It allows the client to interact, even if it is only a short greeting.

Music can act as a timekeeper, aiding the individual with muscle movement by stimulating the brain's motor systems. Rhythmic sounds tapped to or listened to in a song can help the individual with repetition and movement. Rhythmic sound aids the brain to time and sequence movement properly. Music therapy can involve rhythmic drumming, singing, instrument playing, or listening to recorded music.

Music has been found to improve orientation, reduce pain, ease stress and depression, and decrease memory loss. It also increases personal empowerment and emotional empathy, stimulates the immune system, and leads to faster recovery and rehabilitation. Music therapy can be used in conjunction with conventional therapeutic and medical interventions.

You can sing familiar songs to help elicit speech intelligibility and word recall such as:

You Are My Sunshine
Happy Birthday to You
America the Beautiful

Ask family members for a list of the individual's favorite songs or musical preferences.

The Oral-Facial Therapy Exercise Book
2021 Edition

Chapter 6: Neck Exercises

Head Massage

As an extension to the laryngeal, neck, and tinnitus acupressure points, it is effective to massage the head for an overall release of head, neck, and facial musculature.

Embrace the back of your head with both hands, using stretched open palms and fingers. With mild to moderate pressure, grab your head with your fingers and pull them inward towards your palms. Massage your scalp and underlying musculature. Continue for 3 to 5 massage cycles (one cycle equals the time it takes you to pull your hands slowly inward).

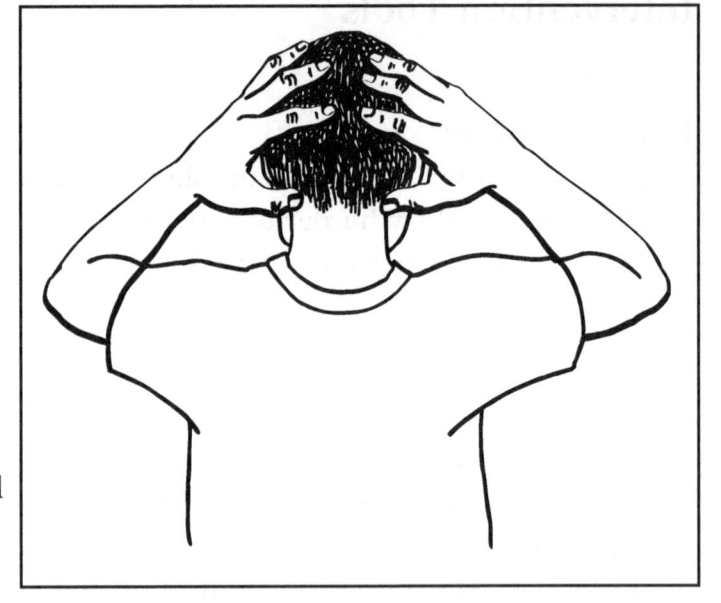

Then continue the massage by moving your hands so one is on each side of your head. Perform for 3 to 5 massage cycles.

As you massage, ask:

- Is the area sensitive to the touch?
- Is the underlying musculature stiff and cord-like?
- Does it hurt when pressure is applied?
- Is it a relief to provide touch to the area?

If the answer is *yes* to any of these questions, it is an indication of muscle irritation and/or tense musculature. Slowly work into the stiffness and apply pressure that is tolerable. Avoid any area that appears bruised.

Back of Neck Release

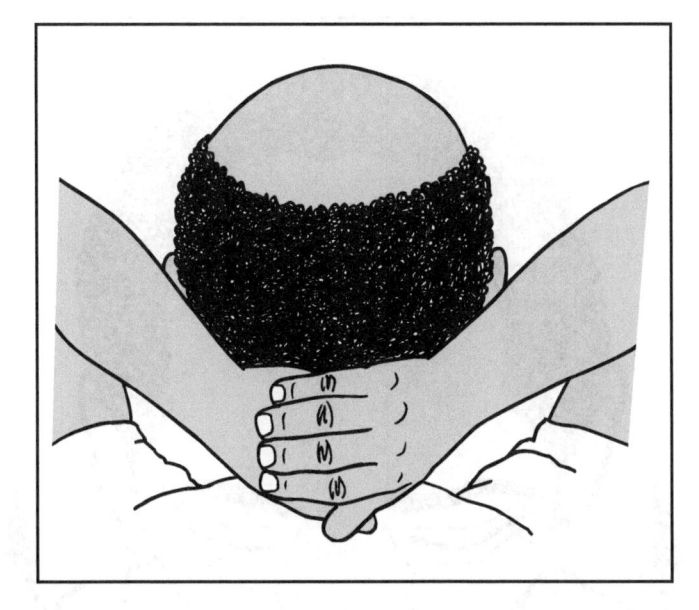

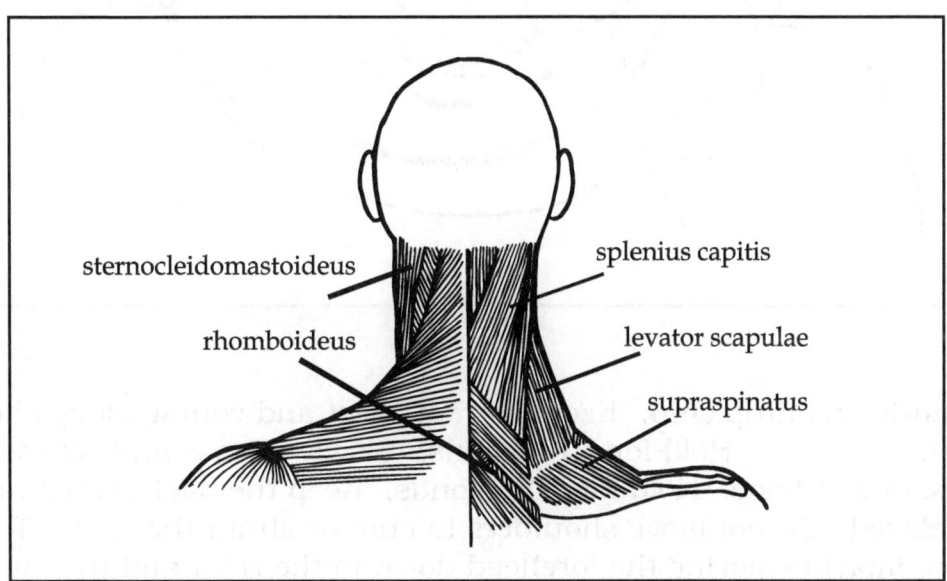

Chapter 6, *continued*

Place the open palm of one hand around the back of the neck as low as possible (where the neck meets the shoulders) and squeeze. Alternate with the other hand. To strengthen the squeeze, use both hands, covering one with the other. Work your hands up the neck. Repeat once.

Benefits

- releases the neck at the upper back to reduce restricted range of motion and pain
- increases range of motion of the head

The Oral-Facial Therapy Exercise Book
2021 Edition

Copyright © 2021

Head Down Lateral Neck Stretch

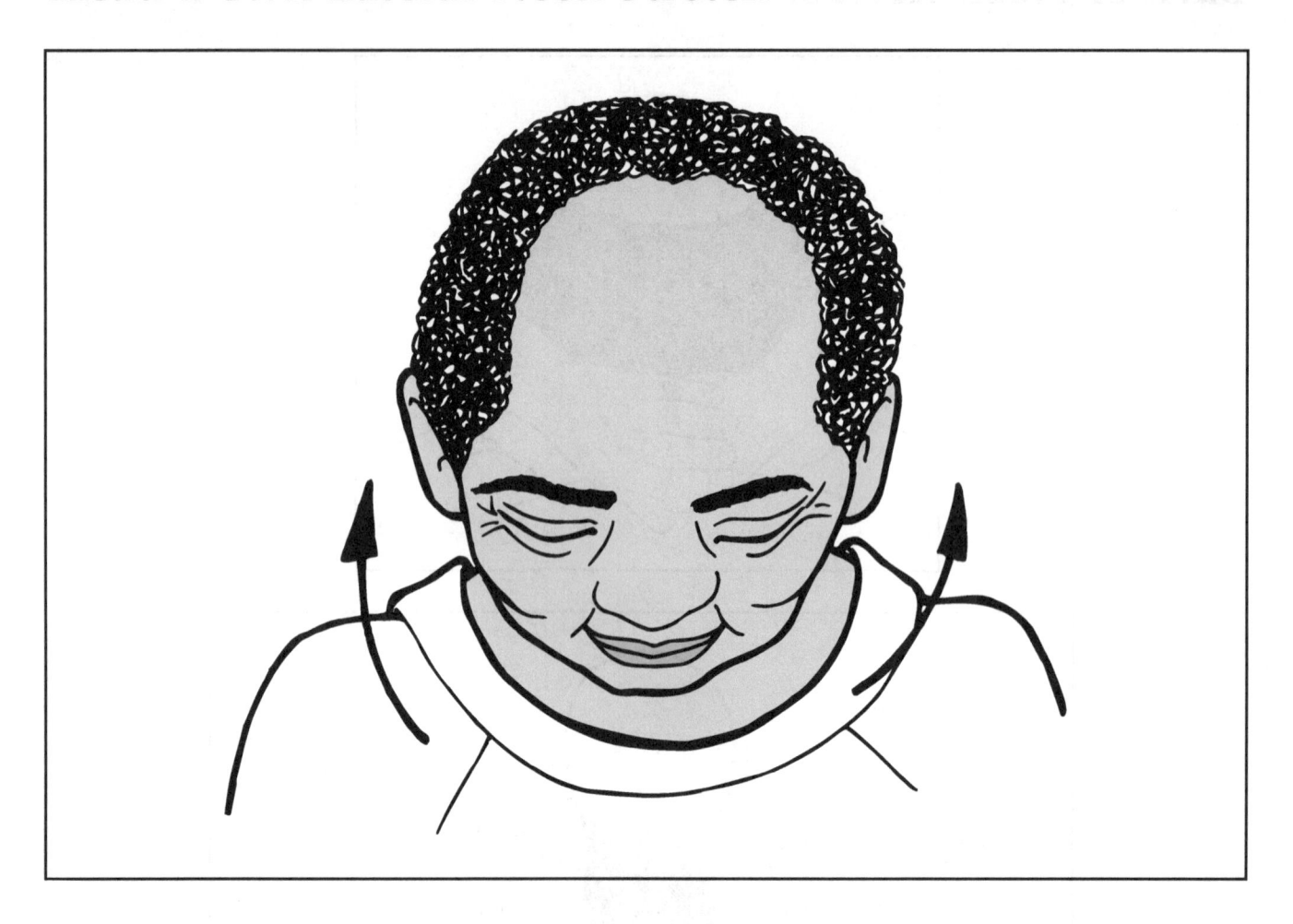

Chapter 6, continued

Close jaw gently and drop chin. Keep chin on chest and course along chest to right shoulder bone (clavicle). Hold for 10 seconds. Slowly release and course back toward left shoulder bone. Hold for 10 seconds. Keep the back straight and shoulders relaxed. Do not move shoulders to chin or strain the neck. To avoid neck tension, imagine moving the forehead down to the right and then to the left.

Benefit

- stretches, tones, and improves range of motion of rear neck

Lateral Neck Stretch

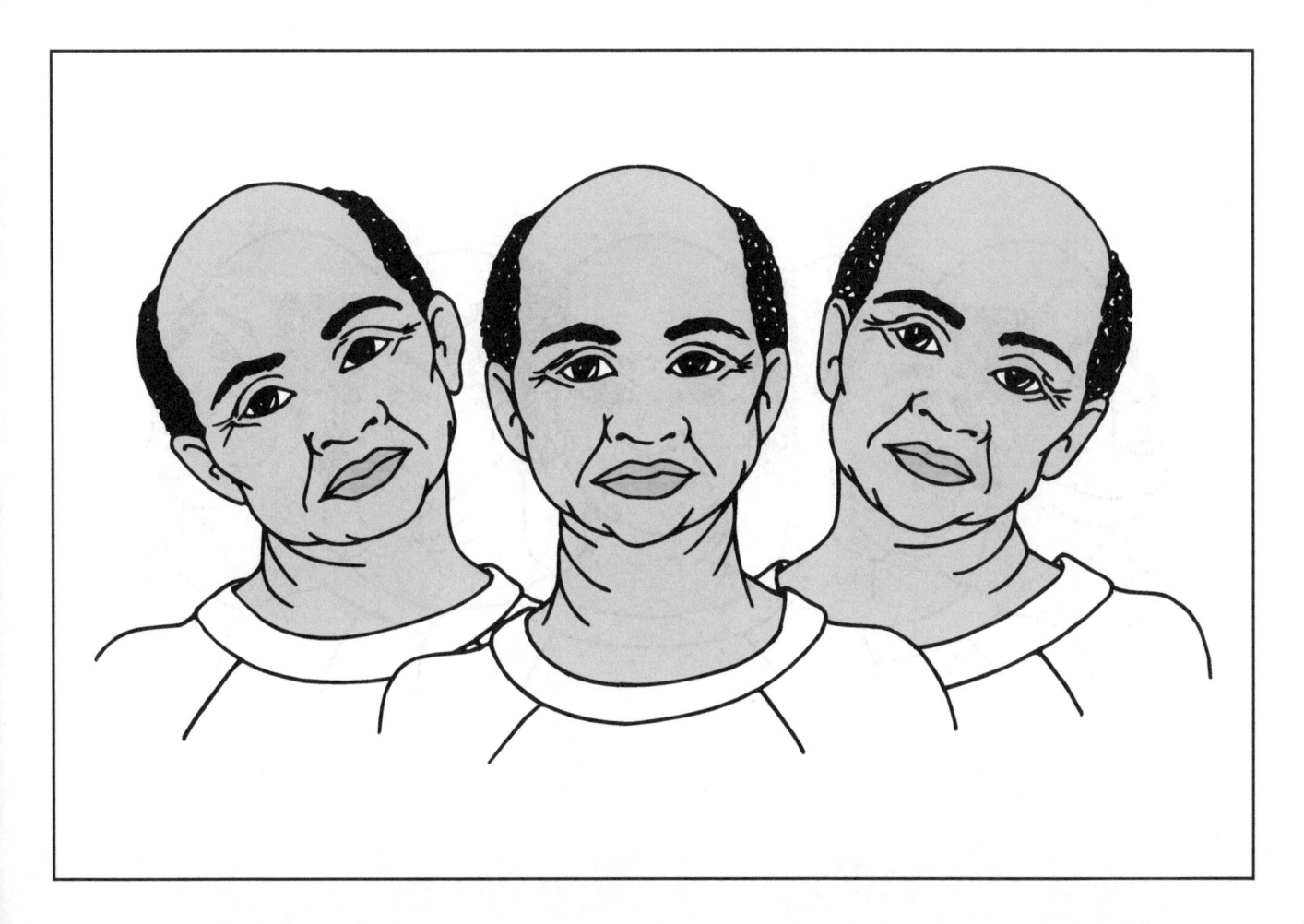

Chapter 6, continued

Look straight ahead throughout exercise. Bend neck so that right ear goes toward right shoulder. Go as far as you can without discomfort and/or raising the right shoulder. Hold for 10 seconds. The goal is for a gentle stretch of the neck, not the shoulder. Keep back upright and shoulders down. Gently move back over to the left side. Hold for 10 seconds, bending neck so that left ear goes toward left shoulder. Keep neck muscles relaxed during exercise.

Benefit

- stretches, tones, and improves range of motion of lateral neck

Extended Lateral Neck Stretch

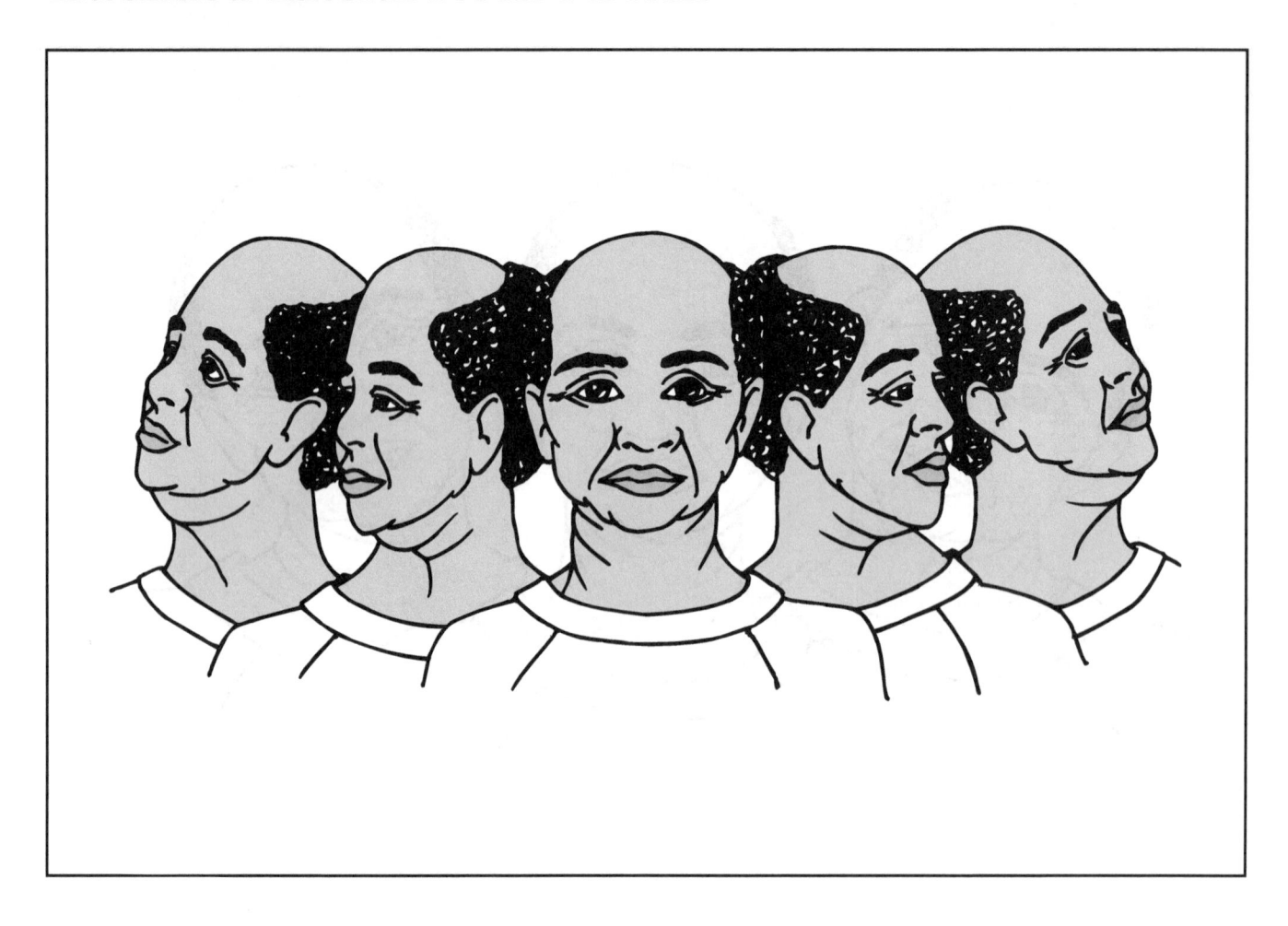

Chapter 6, continued

Sit upright in a chair with the shoulders back and the back straight. **No muscles should be strained or tensed.**

Rest arms at your side and look straight ahead. Slowly turn head to right. Continue turning your head only to the right. Stretch to full extension, but not to pain point. Hold for 10 seconds. Slowly move head around to full left. Hold.

Incorrect form can result in shoulders and waist twisting which gives minimal stretch to the neck. To increase range of motion, tilt head up to the ceiling when at far right and then when at far left.

Benefit

○ stretches, tones, and improves range of motion of lateral neck

Neck and Back Stretch

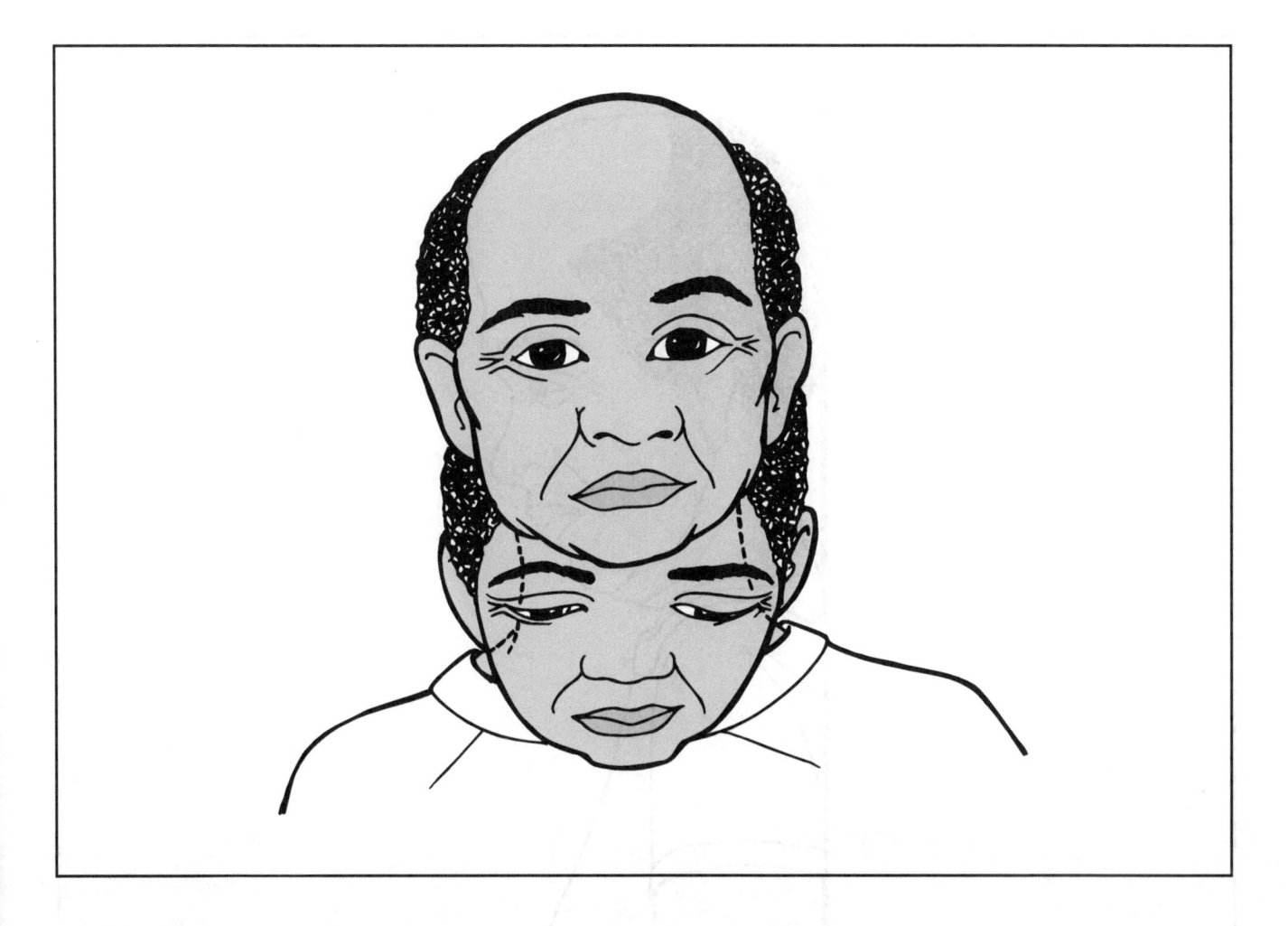

Chapter 6, continued

Look straight ahead. Bend head and neck down toward knees. Keep back straight and shoulders back. Hold for 10 seconds.

To increase complexity, hold neck and head down and slowly bend from the waist to full extension. Go as far as possible without pain. Hold for 5 to 10 seconds as tolerated.

Benefit

- stretches, tones, and improves range of motion of posterior musculature of neck and back

The Oral-Facial Therapy Exercise Book
2021 Edition

Rear Neck Stretch

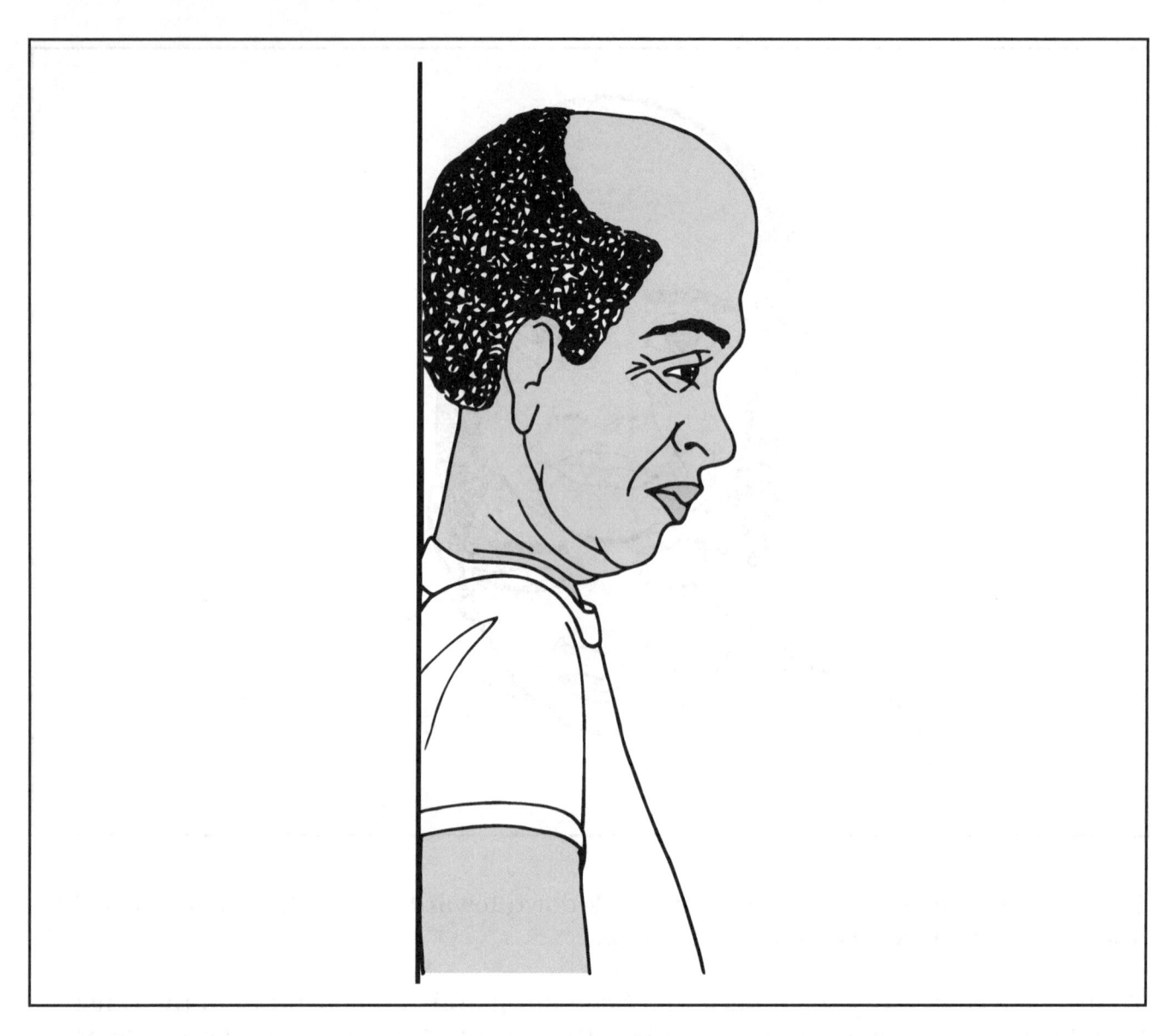

Chapter 6, continued

Remove any items (e.g., hair clasps) which could interfere with the full extension of the neck. Stand with back, head, and shoulders (if possible) touching a wall. (This exercise may also be performed while sitting with the back to a wall or lying in bed with no pillow.)

Push the back of the neck into the wall as close to the wall as possible with head and back touching the wall. Begin by holding for 10 seconds, eventually building up to 30 seconds. Hold.

Benefit

- stretches rear neck musculature

Chapter 7:
Voice and Soft Palate Exercises

Vocal Quality

Note: Schedule an evaluation with an otolaryngologist before beginning any voice therapy. Vocal dysfunction has many etiologies and it's important to rule out any medical involvement.

Breathy vocal quality can result from weakened vocal fold closure. Strong closure is necessary for the vibration which produces sound. Whispered speech, which doesn't involve vibration of the vocal folds, can arise out of habit or fatigue. Whispering is an inappropriate means of voicing because the vocal folds are held apart. To improve vocal quality, adduction exercises for the vocal folds are beneficial. These exercises will encourage the closure and strengthening of the vocal folds and surrounding arytenoid cartilage. The vocal folds work like a hand-held fan. They are connected on one end and open on the other. Voicing takes place as air passes through the vocal folds. The vocal folds then adduct, or come closely together. Vibrations on the edge of the vocal folds occur when air passes through. Sound is then produced. Without this sound source, there is no voicing.

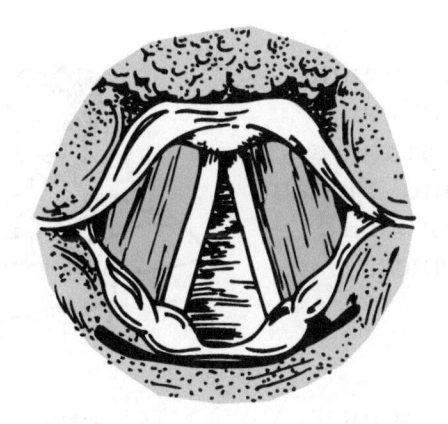

open vocal cords   **closed vocal cords**

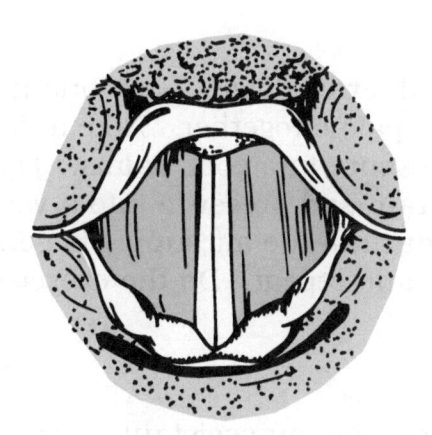

The vocal cord adduction exercises on the next page can be performed in three ways. Each will provide resistance to adduct the vocal folds as well as to strengthen the vocal mechanism. Strengthened vocal fold adduction will aid in protection of the air passageway, thereby preventing aspiration. These exercises will help the client increase loudness and vocal quality. It's important to practice at least three times daily to achieve the maximum benefits from the exercises.

The Oral-Facial Therapy Exercise Book
2021 Edition

Vocal Fold Adduction Exercises

1. Sit in a free-standing chair. Grab onto the sides and take a deep breath. Lift up on the seat while pushing your body onto the chair. Try to make a loud vocal grunting or straining noise while exerting pressure. The pressure will cause your vocal folds to close, and therefore, give you more strength to push yourself down into the chair.

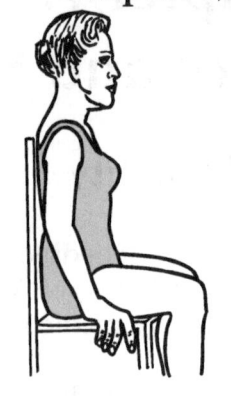

   Sustain the vocal grunt as long as your air supply lasts. Rest for approximately 15 seconds and repeat. Do the exercise 10 times, holding each one as long as possible. Each time, work toward a more physical effort and a louder grunt.

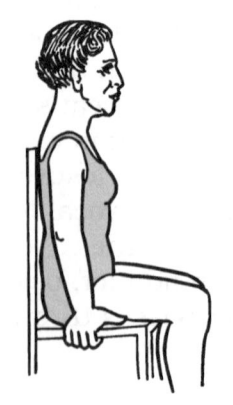

2. Sit, stand, or lie down. Positioning isn't important. Put both palms together. Take a deep breath and exert pressure into your palms. Try to exert the same strain and pressure into a vocal grunt. Sustain the grunt until the air supply is gone. Rest for 15 seconds and repeat. Do the exercise 10 times.

3. Sit across from an assistant. Have the assistant grasp your right palm (or whichever is your strongest hand and arm) with her right palm. Have the assistant press against your palm. Match the pressure with your palm. This will create the pressure necessary to cause the vocal folds to come together (adduct). Produce loud, strained vocal grunting. Rest for 15 seconds and repeat. Do the exercise 10 times, sustaining pressure with maximum force as long as your air supply lasts.

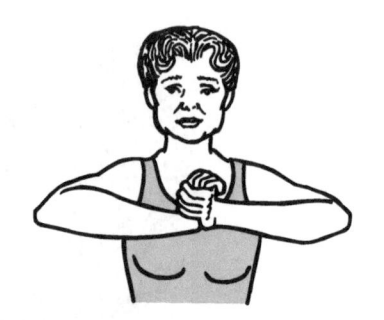

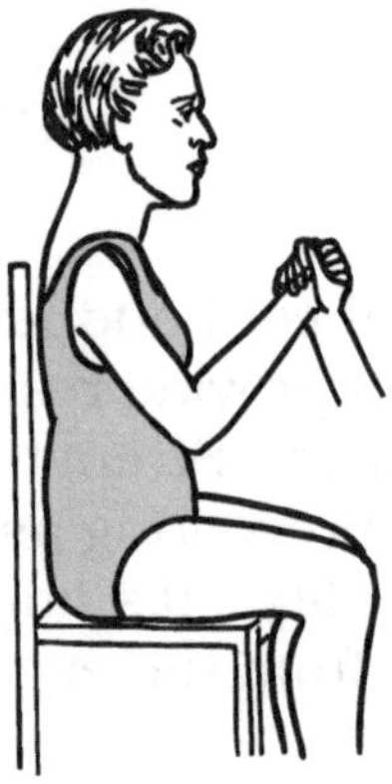

Palatal Stretch

Chapter 7, continued

Clients exhibiting vocal strain or hard glottal onset are good candidates for laryngeal relaxation. Both vocal strain and hard glottal onset can cause hyperadduction of the vocal folds. The rule of thumb for laryngeal relaxation is LESS AIR, LESS PRESSURE, and LESS VOLUME. This means there is less expiratory effect with less laryngeal involvement at a low vocal intensity.

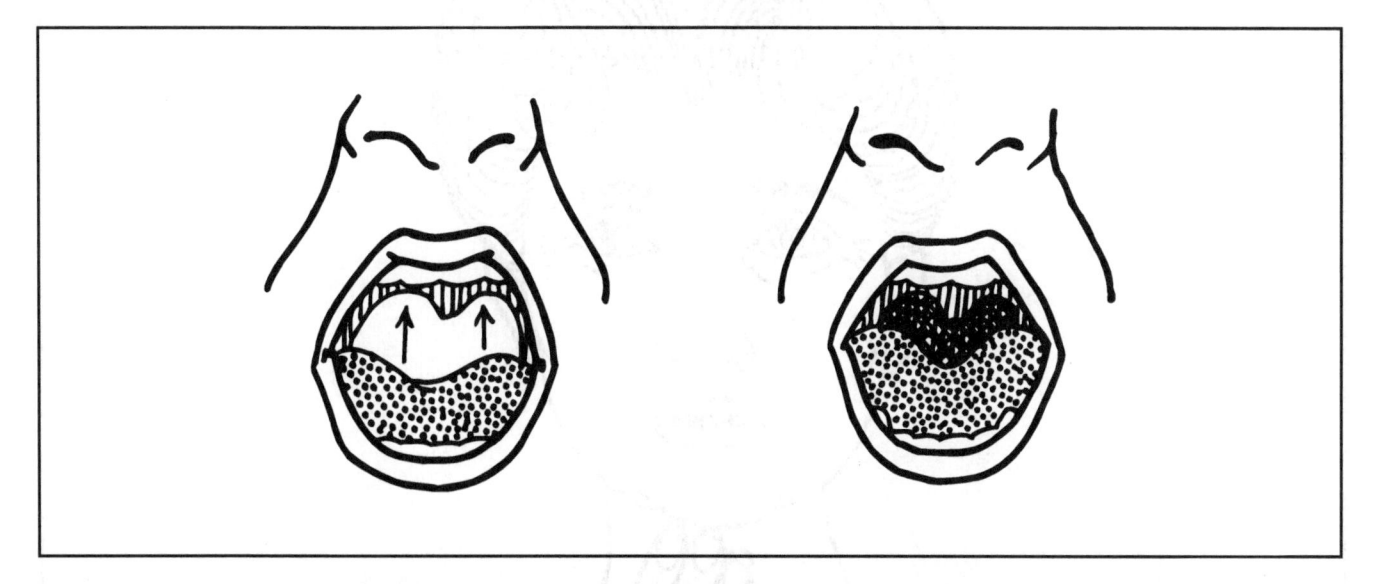

Have the client open her jaw wide and begin a large, forced inhalation-phase yawn. Encourage her to hold the yawn, stretching the soft palate up. Have her push down the back of her tongue as if to make room for a large ball. The client should stretch the left side of the back of her tongue, then the right side. Before the client releases the full-yawn position, she should stretch both sides in an attempt to enlarge the opening in the back of the mouth and pharynx. Complete the exercise with a hard, dry swallow.

The goal of this exercise is to encourage the client to tolerate more and more stimulation to the area so food can be safely transmitted through the hypopharynx comfortably and safely. Many individuals have a very sensitive gag reflex that diminishes their ability to handle certain foods (e.g., hard foods, dry foods, large boluses). The gag reflex will diminish with stretching as it makes the area less sensitive. If a client gags, reassure her that she is all right. Remind her to breathe through her nose.

Benefits

- improves vocal quality by stretching and toning the palate for improved resonance in the oral/pharyngeal/nasal cavity
- relaxes palate and throat musculature to reduce discomfort during swallowing

Tactile Voicing

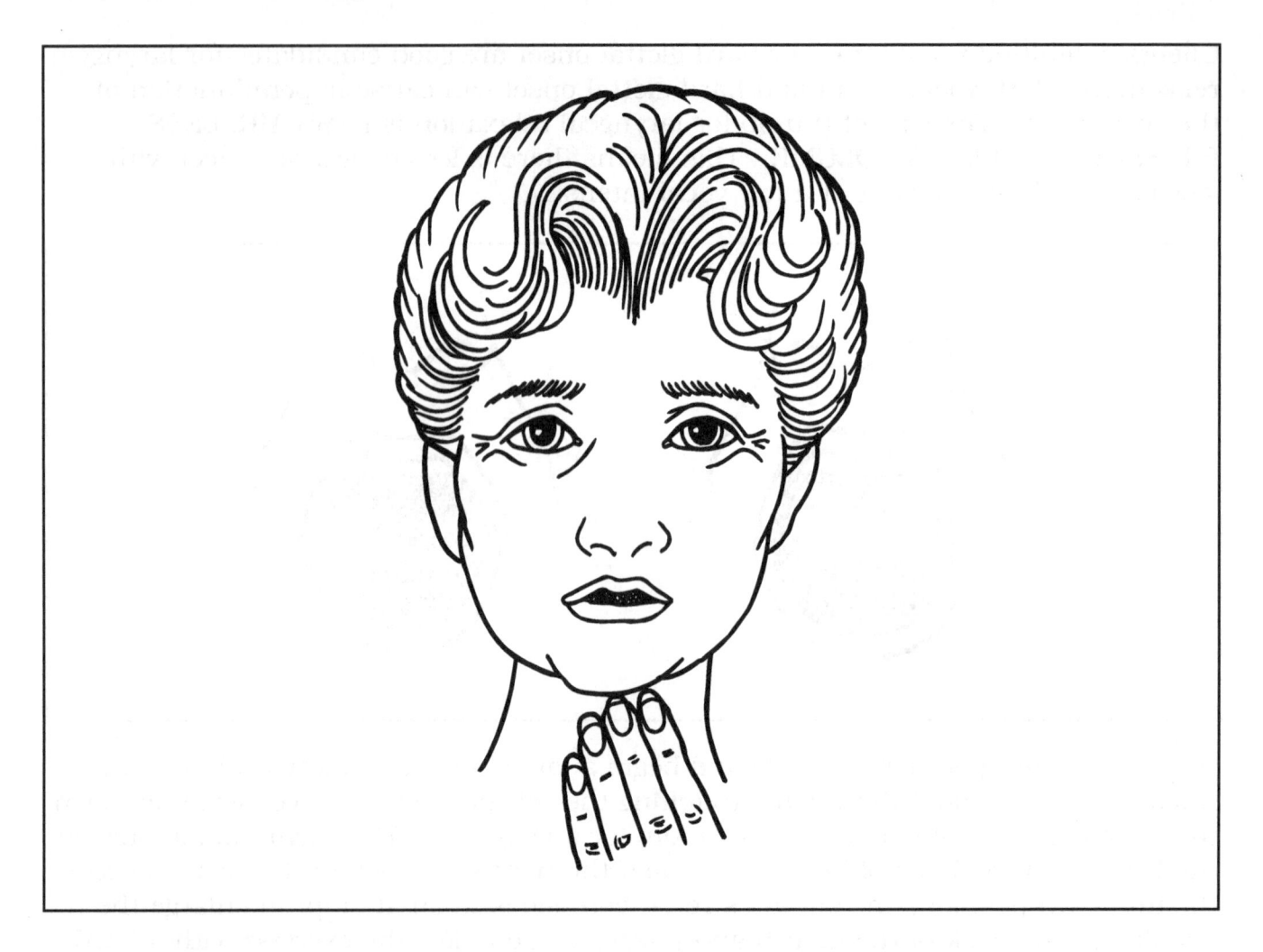

Chapter 7, continued

Place the palm of your hand on your therapist's throat to feel the vibration of sound during voicing. Then move your palm to your own throat. Inhale deeply. Say, "ah" as you exhale to feel the vibration. Go back and forth from your own throat to the therapist's throat.

Note: Increase loudness as needed to help the client feel the vibration.

Benefits

- teaches individual voice onset
- improves adduction of vocal folds for voicing

Oral Resonance

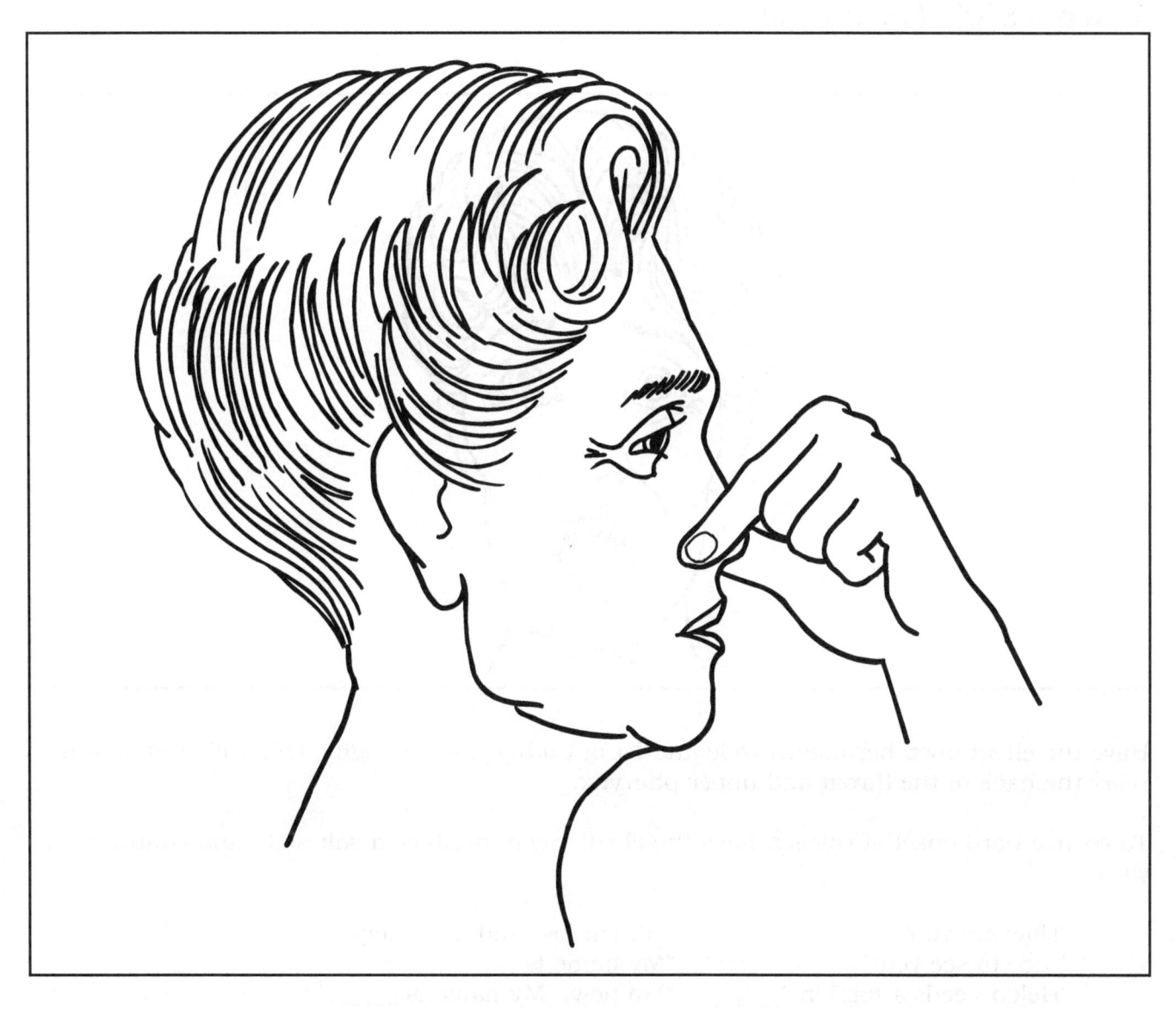

Chapter 7, continued

Pinch your nostrils securely so you breathe through your mouth (orally). Say, "ah" as you exhale. Repeat. As pressure on your nostrils is gradually lessened, try to maintain the "ah" as you exhale. Repeat with other vowels ("ee," "I," "o," "oo," "u").

Note: A nose clip may be used to free hand from face during this exercise.

Benefit

- improves oral resonance and oral voicing

Yawn – Sigh Technique

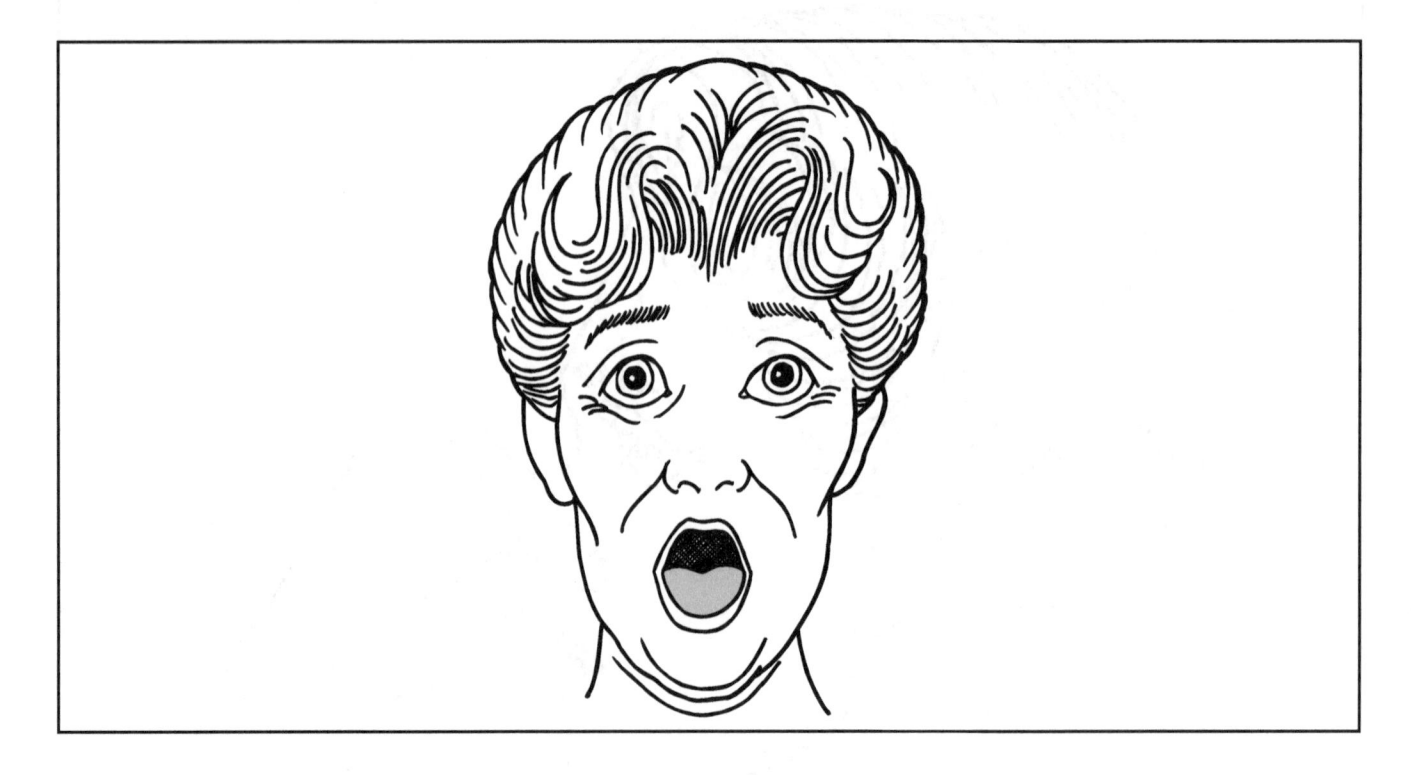

Have the client open her mouth wide and let out a big yawn or sigh. This will stretch and relax the back of the throat and upper pharynx.

To reduce hard onset of voicing, have the client yawn, produce a soft sigh, and continue with:

"How are you?" "Hi, I'm lost and need help."
"Nice to see you." "My name is ____."
"Helen needs a napkin." "I'm new. My name is ____."

Increase the complexity with vowel-initiated sentences.

Add the chewing technique (i.e., move jaw during word production). This will release the jaw and soften the initial tension produced on phonation.

Chapter 7, *continued*

Exercises for Sustaining Voice

These exercises are provided to help initiate and sustain voicing. Begin with Exercise 1 and proceed through Exercise 4.

Exercise 1

Have the client start with easy onset, make a glottal fry or hard onset, and then finish with easy onset again. Use /h/-initiated vowel productions followed by vowel-only productions.

    hah → ah   ho → o   hih → ih
    hee → ee   hoo → oo   heh → eh
    hi → i

hah ———————————————————————— ah

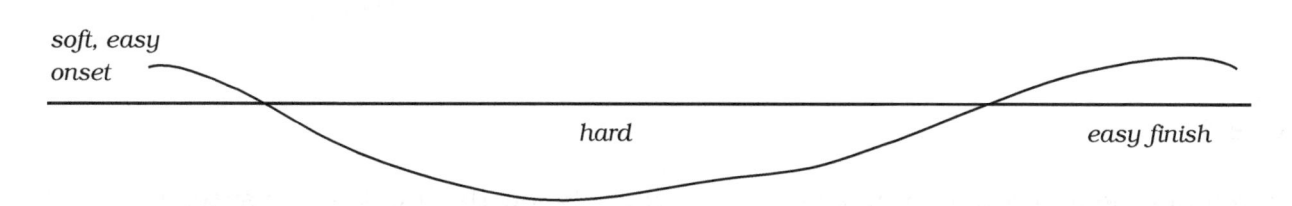

soft, easy onset ⋯⋯ *hard* ⋯⋯ *easy finish*

Exercise 2

Model glottal attack or hard onset of voicing so the client sees the opposite of easy onset. Show the increased strain to the neck. Draw a line showing the high degree of tension which characterizes a hard onset of phonation.

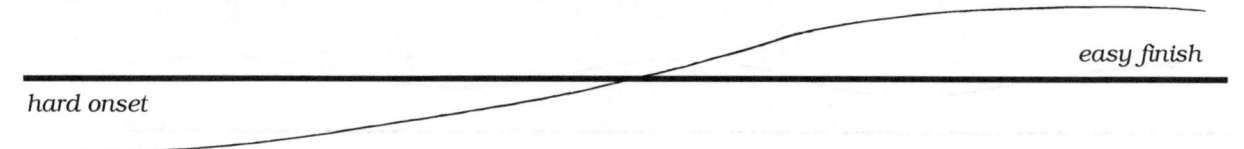

hard onset ⋯⋯ *easy finish*

Have the individual practice reducing muscle tightness, reducing the amount of air used, and reducing loudness. Encourage the client to follow the line up, lowering her voice as well as decreasing the effort it takes to make herself heard. Remind her not to whisper, but to just talk slowly and effortlessly. Use analogies like the ones described below to make the transition from hard onset to soft onset voicing.

- Start out talking like you are talking to someone across the room. Now gradually soften your voice so as not to wake a baby sleeping next to you.

- Turn the volume of the loud speaker down till you can barely hear the message being broadcast.

- Speak as if very excited and nervous. Soothe into a voice of someone who is very reassuring, calming, and peaceful.

Chapter 7, continued

Exercises for Sustaining Voice, continued

Exercise 3

Then have the client begin with easy onset using yawn/sigh or words beginning with /h/. Have her go below the line to glottal fry or hard, tense speech production to see and feel the opposite.

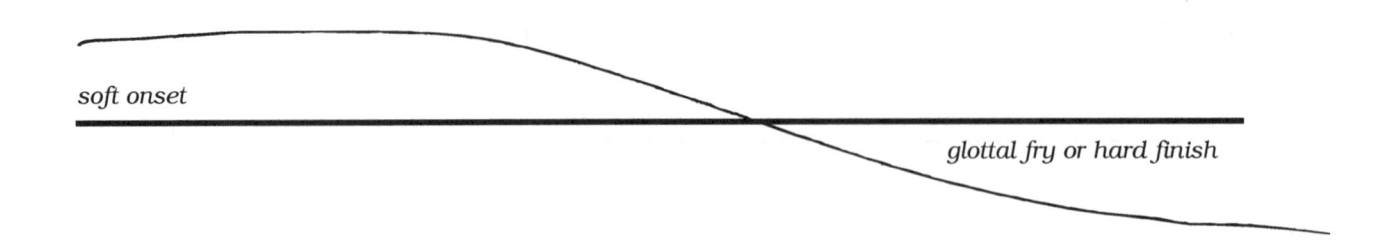

soft onset

glottal fry or hard finish

Exercise 4

Lastly, remind the individual not to go below the line. Below the line is tense speech or glottal fry productions. Sustain flow of production through a decrease in neck and laryngeal tension, a reduction in the force or amount of airflow, and a decrease in loudness.

Increase complexity of productions with words and sentences. Start easy, continue easy, and end with easy flow of voicing.

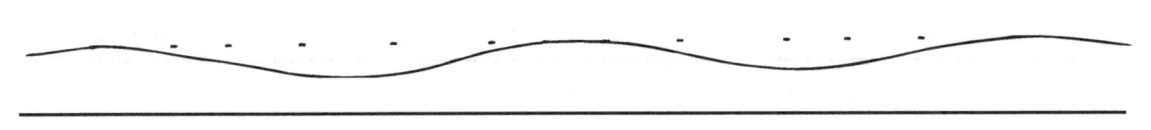

sustained voicing without going below the line into glottal fry or hard-voiced productions

Chapter 7, *continued*

Phrasing

Clear articulation involves precise movement of the tongue, lips, jaw, and vocal folds with respiratory support for voicing. Any impairment or atrophy of these articulators can cause:

- slurred speech
- omission of sounds in words
- mumbling
- jumbling

Clients having difficulty articulating (e.g., those who have had a stroke, neurological involvement, Parkinson's disease) will begin to blend words together, making one long unintelligible stream of sounds or simplifying words. For example, a client might say, "tawber milkake" instead of "strawberry milk shake." The simplification occurs because the client is unable to make the quick changes in tongue, lip, and jaw placement necessary in rapid conversation. In addition, she will often try to speak even faster because of poor respiratory support. The client will probably run out of air due to shallow inspiration, improper phrasing, or weakened vocal folds.

Training to improve articulation in words, phrases, and sentences, along with instruction in proper breath support will produce clearer speech.

Box Speech

Box Speech is a technique that teaches the client to say each word without jumbling. Jumbling occurs when a client speaks unintelligibly due to poor air support. By putting each word in a box, the client learns to finish one word before beginning the next. This technique will produce louder, clearer speech.

Ask the client to say one word only, starting with the first box word on the next page, "I". Have her inhale and say the word as she exhales. Then have the client repeat this step for each word in the sentence. It is helpful to use the circular breathing chart, described in the Breathing and Visualization section of this book to remember to inhale and upon the exhale vocalize the word in the box. Initially speech is slow because of the new air supply for each word.

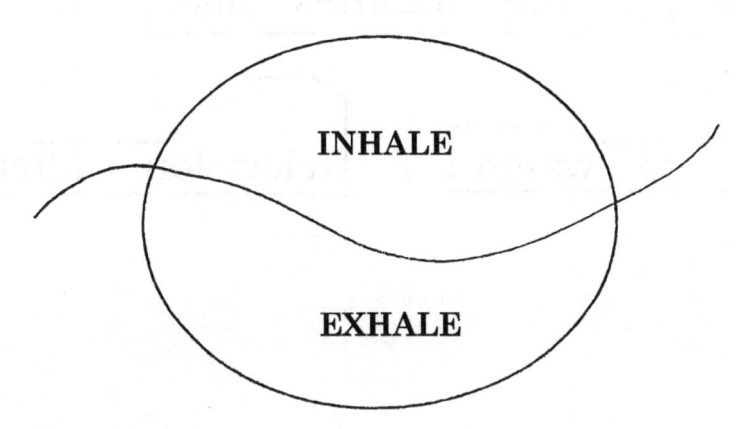

INHALE

EXHALE

Chapter 7, *continued*

| I | | would | | like | | a | | drink. |

The next stage involves bisyllabic words. Use a full inhalation before each word and exhale as the word is spoken. If the client has extra air remaining after producing the word, tell her to exhale the rest and start each word with a fresh inhalation.

| baseball | | listen | | hungry | | cellar | | paper |

The goal of Box Speech is to expand the number of syllables and words per box while maintaining individual sound production and replenishing air supply between boxes.

| And so | | it goes. |

Continue to increase the complexity of the words in Box Speech. Remind the client to produce all the sounds and to replenish air between the boxes. Give the client time to speak clearly.

| Take the time to | | speak clearly. |

Have the client look at the height of the box for each word as she is reading to reflect changes in intonation and pitch. (Note: Higher line indicates a raise in pitch. The slashes indicate a place to take a breath.)

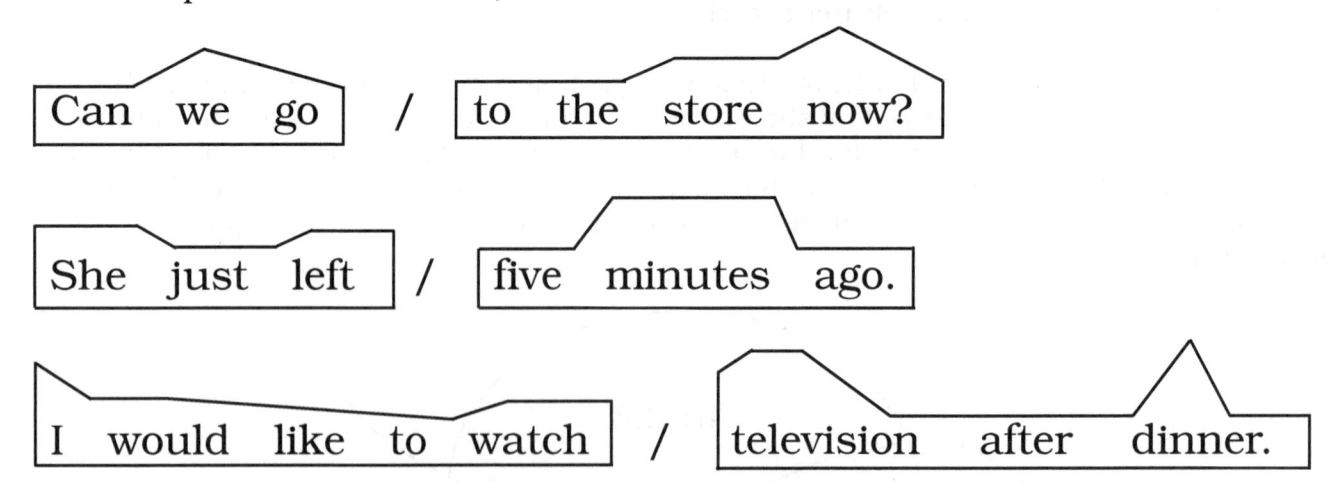

| Can we go | / | to the store now? |

| She just left | / | five minutes ago. |

| I would like to watch | / | television after dinner. |

The Oral-Facial Therapy Exercise Book
2021 Edition

Chapter 7, *continued*

As the client phrases properly, stopping to replenish air supply and using intonation as a means of segmenting speech, introduce more complex sentences at the paragraph level. The paragraph below will provide practice for the client. The slashes indicate breathing points. Have the client mark her own breathing points before reading the story aloud from a magazine or book. Then encourage the client to go through another story without the written cues.

The other day/ I decided to take my dog, Sadie,/ for a walk./ She was reluctant to go outside/ because it was cold and dreary./ I tried all the usual ploys./ What else could I do/ but pick up her little 12-pound/ furry body/ and start walking?/ I set her down a couple of houses from mine,/ hoping she had changed her mind/ and decided it wasn't such a bad idea/ to take a walk on a brisk afternoon./ Sadie looked at me with the sorriest brown eyes/ and refused to budge./ I promised to walk straight back home,/ but she wouldn't move./ I ended up carrying her back./ While carrying her, I wondered/ who was the doggone master of whom!

The Oral-Facial Therapy Exercise Book
2021 Edition

Shoulder Shrug

If the individual is experiencing relatively high clavicular (collarbone), shoulder, or chest rise during breathing, perform this exercise to bring the breath down. It will free the voice by reducing the tension created during inhalation and voiced exhalation. The exercise releases the neck, jaw, collarbone, and ribs to allow the breath to expand. It opens the voice and produces a relaxing and centering effect. The shoulder shrug starts with exaggerated tension and shows the individual the opposite, the release of tension. The goal is to have the client focus on lower intake of each breath, away from the shoulders and clavicle.

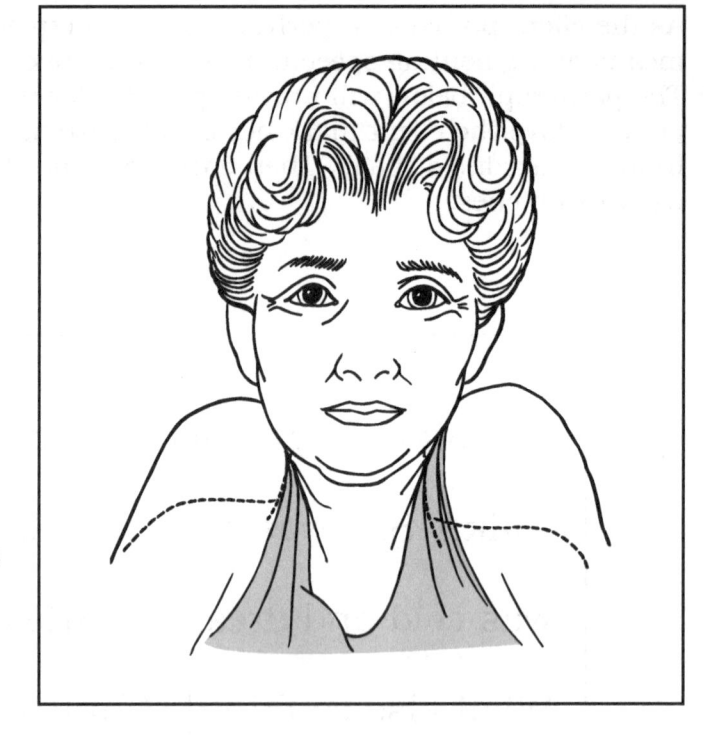

If possible, have the individual sit upright in a chair with good support (e.g., pillows in the back and/or on the sides). The client should be comfortable and not holding herself up by balancing her upper body. If the individual is lying down, have her sit up as much as possible. Do not use excessive pillows to raise her head as this can bend the neck and force the head forward. Use one pillow which allows the head to tilt slightly. If the bed is adjustable, tilt the head portion of the bed up too. If the bed doesn't adjust, support the individual from the waist up with a wedge or pillows so that the head and neck are not overly bent.

Once the client is comfortable, have her raise her shoulders up to her ears and take a deep breath. Have the client count aloud to 5 as she drops her shoulders and releases air with each number. When the shoulders have come to the optimal resting point (down and relaxed), have the individual take a deep breath. Watch that the client does not raise her shoulders. This deep breath is taken in from where the shoulders left off in the lower position. Then have the client count from 6 to 10, releasing air with each number as the shoulders continue to drop. This will show the client quite naturally how to take in the breath from the lower chest or diaphragm without bringing attention to it. Repeat once.

Then have the client breathe in more deeply (i.e., to the pelvis) without raising her shoulders. Tell her to keep her shoulders down and to exhale on the count of 11 to 15. Repeat, having the client take another deep breath (i.e., to the knees) and count aloud from 16 to 20. The voice will free up and may crack intermittently. The client may try to hold on to the tension or inappropriate voicing. Let her know that the new voice which is more resonant and velvety is appropriate. Do not encourage deepening of the pitch or a forced exhalation. The breath will merely fall out. The individual's attention is focused lower in the body as she breathes down farther and farther.

Chapter 7, *continued*

Lowering the Resonance and Carriage of the Voice

This exercise is beneficial to clients who have a nasal, throaty, crackling, pubescent, and/or falsetto voice. It allows the person to begin voicing in the chest.

Have the individual put her hand on her chest and after taking a deep breath of air, vocalize /ah/. Allow the hand to absorb the vibration. Then have her move her hand to her throat to feel the vibration of the /ah/ at the point of the vocal folds. Have her move her hand back down to the chest and repeat. The airflow or physical effort may be too excessive. If so, have the client place her hand on her chest and try:

○ a quieter, softer voice

○ a high note that goes to a low note

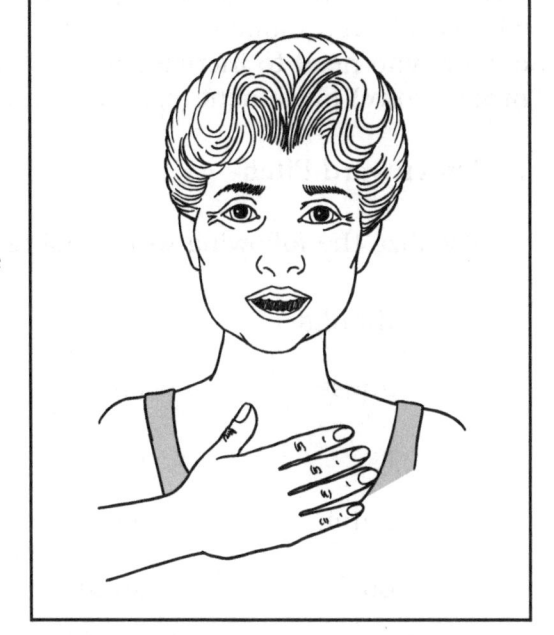

○ bending over at the waist and releasing the /ah/ without shoulder and neck tension restriction.

The vibration felt in the hand will slowly increase as it is generated by the open resonating chamber of the chest. This will decrease head or nasal resonance that is excessive and will give the individual a voice that sounds more from the body. A natural, relaxed type of sound will emerge.

○ increasing from /ah/ to /nah/ to /gah/ and then to /sah/. The client can then move to any words and sentences, maintaining the vowel vibration in the chest. This sound is to be naturally produced and not created through pressure or a lowering of the pitch.

> Note: Natural pitch tone can be assessed in most normal speakers by asking them to hum. Say, "Hum a note for me, anything that feels natural for you." It is best not to model a hum because the average speaker will just repeat the pitch of your hum.

The Oral-Facial Therapy Exercise Book
2021 Edition

Chapter 7, continued

Vocal Exercises

Exercises 1-6 are step-by-step exercises that are beneficial to improve intonation in clients who speak in a monotone or who have a limited pitch range. Exercise 7 is beneficial for clients who need to increase intensity. Exercise 8 is beneficial for anyone interested in proper vowel placement (e.g., accent reduction, neurological decline, head trauma).

1. **Downward Pitch**

    Vocalize the following words using a downward intonation.

thanks	sod	mute	bite
guess	chime	yet	feed
jig	code	sigh	judge
hatch	gown	palm	blob
book	shun	crown	sick
spoon	much	range	eight
chuck	wheeze	length	neat

2. **Upward Pitch**

    Repeat the word list in number 1, moving pitch upward as in a question.

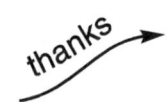

3. **Sentence Intonation Practice: Downward Pitch to Upward Pitch**

    Vary pitch starting with a downward intonation and ending with an upward intonation.

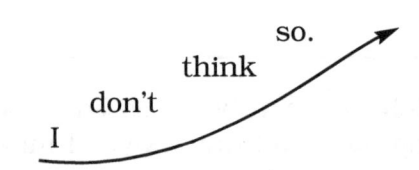

    I don't think so.   No telling what she'll do next.

    Pop goes the weasel.   You can have it; I don't need it.

    She dropped the jug.   She called in sick today.

    Do you like vanilla pudding?   Are the dogs in the house?

    He is as thin as a rail.   Mary makes a good loaf of bread.

Chapter 7, *continued*

4. **Sentence Intonation Practice: Upward Pitch to Downward Pitch**

   Repeat the list in number 3, but start with an upward intonation and finish with a downward intonation. Keep the voice on, using an appropriate amount of air exhaled continuously on voicing.

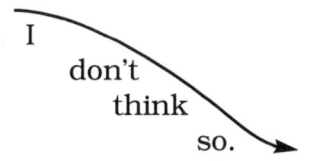

   ```
         I
          don't
              think
                   so.
   ```

5. **Roller Coaster Ride of Intonation**

   Say the following sounds, allowing the intonation to travel freely up and down the average speaking range. You may wish to try this by humming first.

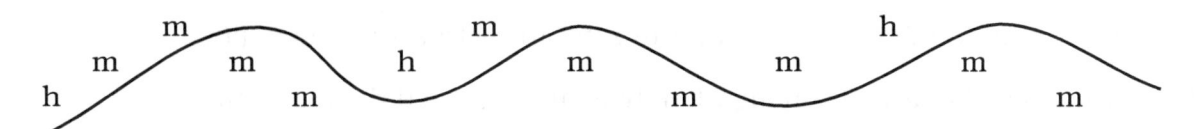

   ```
           m           m                       h
       m       m   h       m           m           m
   h           m               m                       m
   ```

6. **Sticking to my Answer Passage**

   Repeat the passage several times using a different emotional overlay each time.

anger	apathy	immaturity	deceit
hopelessness	frustration	disgust	pain
exhaustion	flat affect	exuberance	sadness
humor	grief	wisdom	insecurity
fear	craziness	worry	sympathy

   Sticking to My Answer

   I have no other answer to that question. It will always be the same answer even if you ask me a million times. My reply will always be the same no matter what, no matter when you ask, unless of course you ask me a different question in a different tone of voice and under different circumstances. Then I may have a different answer, maybe many different answers, and totally fool you and myself. So there.

The Oral-Facial Therapy Exercise Book
2021 Edition

Chapter 7, continued

7. **Increasing Intensity** (loudness)

    Say the first sentence in each pair with average effort. Then say the second sentence with a strong effort (e.g., a loud voice). Take a good breath before each sentence and let yourself really feel the force moving through you on the second sentence.

    > I didn't hear you. What did you say?
    > I am tired. I am really exhausted.
    > You've got it. You've really got it.
    > Take one. Go ahead, take one.
    > I'm resting. Can I get some rest for a minute?

    The following exercises will improve vocal intensity, especially if other factors like apraxia, aphasia, head trauma, or Parkinson's disease are present:

    A. Cough and then attempt to say "ah" with a wide open jaw.

    B. Clear throat loudly. Then attempt to say "ah" with a wide open jaw.

    C. Take a deep breath. Then sigh loudly as if exhausted during exhalation.

    D. Practice saying "hello" loudly with a disconnected telephone. Then practice with a real caller. This works well with clients who are disoriented.

    E. Sing familiar songs. Singing is an effective technique to elicit phonation and expressive speech production in the apraxic patient. You might try:

    > You Are My Sunshine
    > Happy Birthday to You
    > America the Beautiful
    > Take Me Out to the Ball Game

8. **Knowing Proper Vowel Placement** (Standard American English)

    The progression of vowel placement moves from the front to the wide middle, open middle, back, and far back.

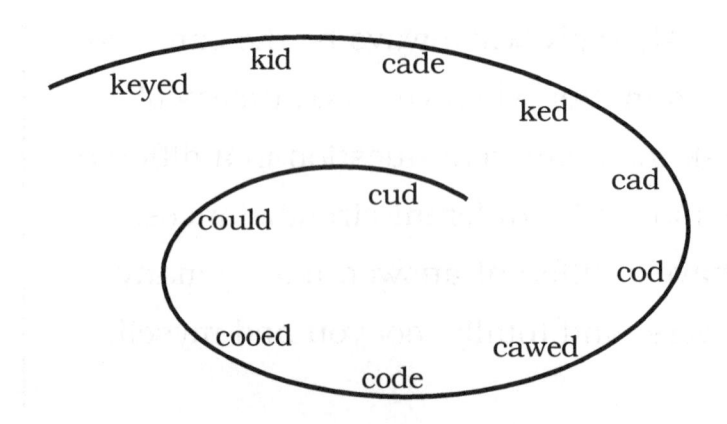

    keyed kid cade
    ked
    cad
    cud
    could
    cod
    cooed cawed
    code

The Oral-Facial Therapy Exercise Book
2021 Edition

Chapter 7, *continued*

Reflux Voice Disorders

Gastroesophageal reflux disease (GERD) extending to the larynx is called *reflux laryngitis*. This problem can frequently be prevented by changes in the timing, type, and amount of food that is eaten. It is best not to recline or go to sleep at least one hour after a meal. Overeating increases the likelihood of recurrent reflux. Food that combines proteins with carbohydrates can often be the culprit for reflux (e.g., meat with potatoes; a sandwich with meat and bread). Also, it is helpful to avoid alcohol, mint, and caffeine. A nutritionist can further recommend a balanced dietary plan.

Treatment for GERD (e.g., dietary changes, lifestyle changes, use of antacids) works for only about 35% of patients because many of them do not follow the regime. Therapy at its best is a cooperative agreement. The individual needs education and follow-up support for optimal intervention success and reassurance that change over time is possible.

Symptoms and laryngeal conditions associated with GERD:

- intermittent or chronic dysphonia
- vocal fatigue
- voice breaks
- chronic throat clearing
- excessive throat mucus
- post-nasal drip
- chronic cough
- dysphagia

At its worst, GERD can be debilitating and life-threatening, causing subglottic stenosis, posterior laryngeal stenosis, arytenoid fixation, carcinoma in a non-smoker, and laryngospasms. Seeing a physician for immediate treatment of this condition is imperative. Medication may be indicated by the physician to treat the symptoms presented. In addition to medical care, individuals have found relief of these symptoms with care from a Homeopathic practitioner and/or Acupuncturist for recommendations of dietary and life style change, change of diet, remedies and treatments.

Begin by getting a voice/larynx and reflux history on the client. Note reoccurrence of nodules, misuse, abuse, congestion, and any symptomology listed above. Report all findings to the referring physician. If the individual has not seen an otolaryngologist, recommend it to the person and/or the primary physician. Follow up with the physician to obtain the results of the diagnostic evaluation.

Dual pH esophageal monitoring measures the amount and frequency of the flow of gastric content flow into the esophagus and larynx over a 24-hour period. This allows for the diagnosis of and proper treatment for reflux laryngitis. Contact a gastrointestinal physician for more information regarding esophageal monitoring.

Soft Palate Closure

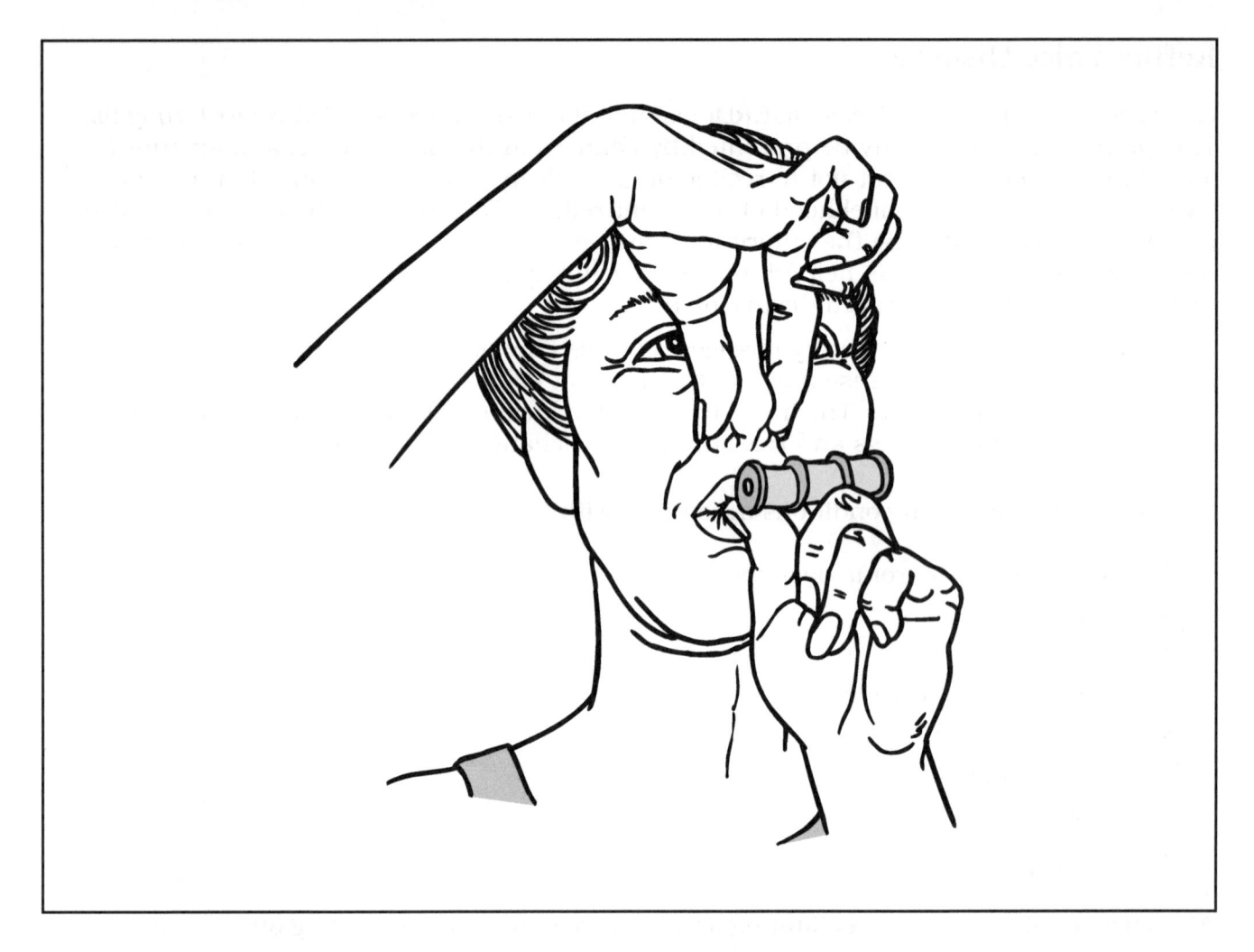

Chapter 7, continued

Blow into a whistle or the long end of a Chewy Tube. Close off the nares to direct the airflow through the oral cavity. Release the nose a little bit at a time to encourage the soft palate to raise. Keep closing and slightly opening the nares and continue to blow hard. Repeat 5 – 10 times.

> Note: To adjust the amount of airflow through the Chewy Tube, close off the sides of the T portion of the tube with index finger and thumb. A whistle will be created.

Benefits

- strengthens soft palate closure for oral voicing
- reduces nasal reflux

Soft Palate Massage

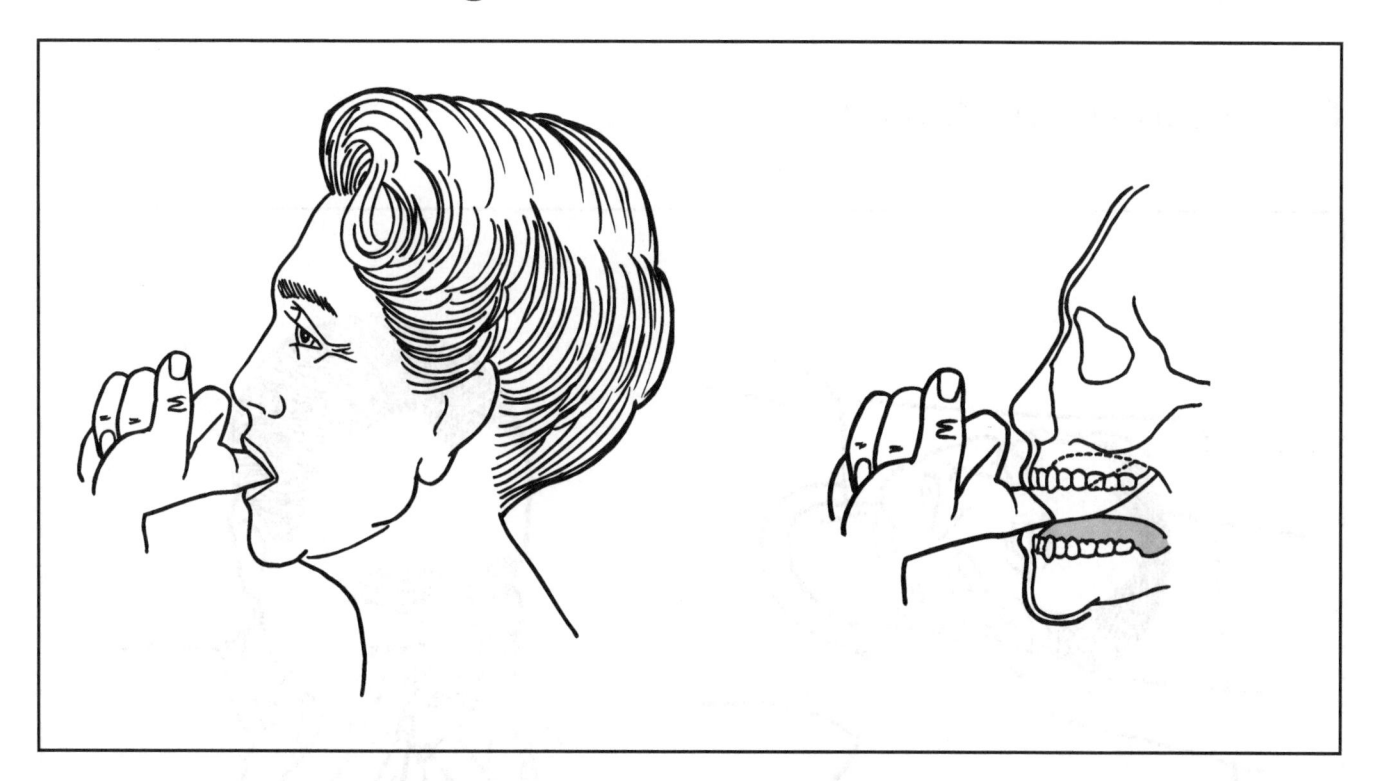

Chapter 7, continued

This exercise is not for everyone. It may cause gagging, vomiting, increased saliva production, or draining of the sinus. It is effective in helping to release the jaw stiffness and tension in the hypopharynx. Enter slowly and press gently on the soft palate (close to the hard palate attachment). Apply pressure as tolerated. When you are able to continue, move the finger along the ridge attachment of the hard palate to the soft palate, applying very light pressure.

Then extend the index finger over to the faucial pillars. Push gently against this area on each side. This area may be massaged without doing the soft palate.

Note: Try this exercise another day if gagging or vomiting occurs.

Benefits

- stretches the soft palate
- reduces gagging
- opens the throat for improved chewing and voicing
- indirectly releases tension in the abdomen

Chapter 8: Cheek Exercises

Cheek and Lip Assist

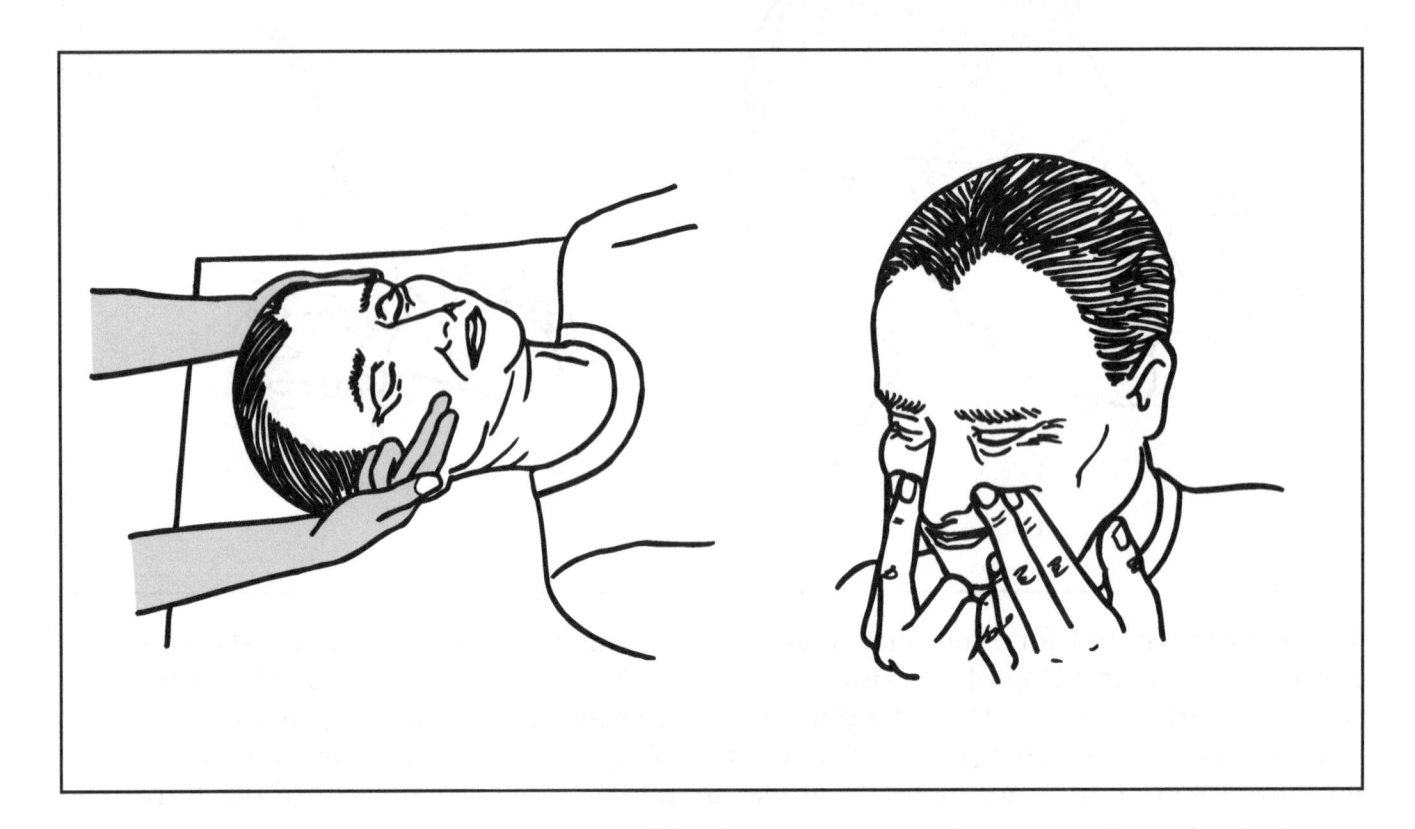

Press fingers upward against the ridge of the cheekbone. These muscles, the zygomaticus major and zygomaticus minor, draw the mouth backward and upward. They are responsible for the expression of pleasure or a good laugh. Work both sides, either one at a time or at the same time. Move in several directions, even if one side is severely weakened or paralyzed.

Benefits

- stretches and tones cheek musculature
- assists in upward motion of cheeks and lips

Top of the Cheekbone

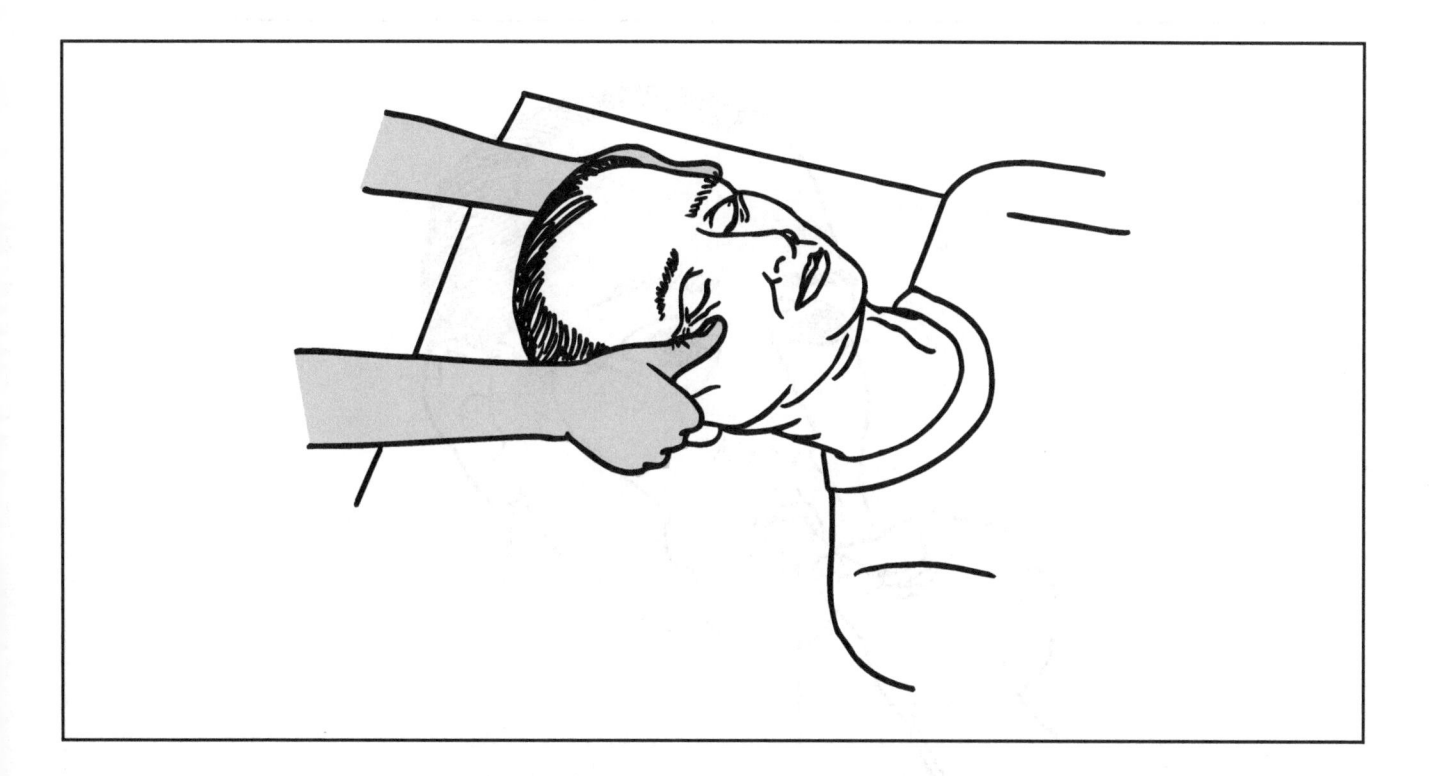

Chapter 8, continued

Press the length of the thumb down on the top ridge of the cheekbone. Hold for about 5 to 10 seconds, rocking the thumb slowly along this line maintaining steady pressure. Repeat on the other side.

Stretch by moving the cheek in several directions. This intervention leaves a warm, alert feeling to the muscle. Make sure to do both sides, even in the case of severe weakness or paralysis.

Benefits

- stretches and tones cheek musculature
- helps to reduce stress and muscle tension

Inner Cheek Strengthener

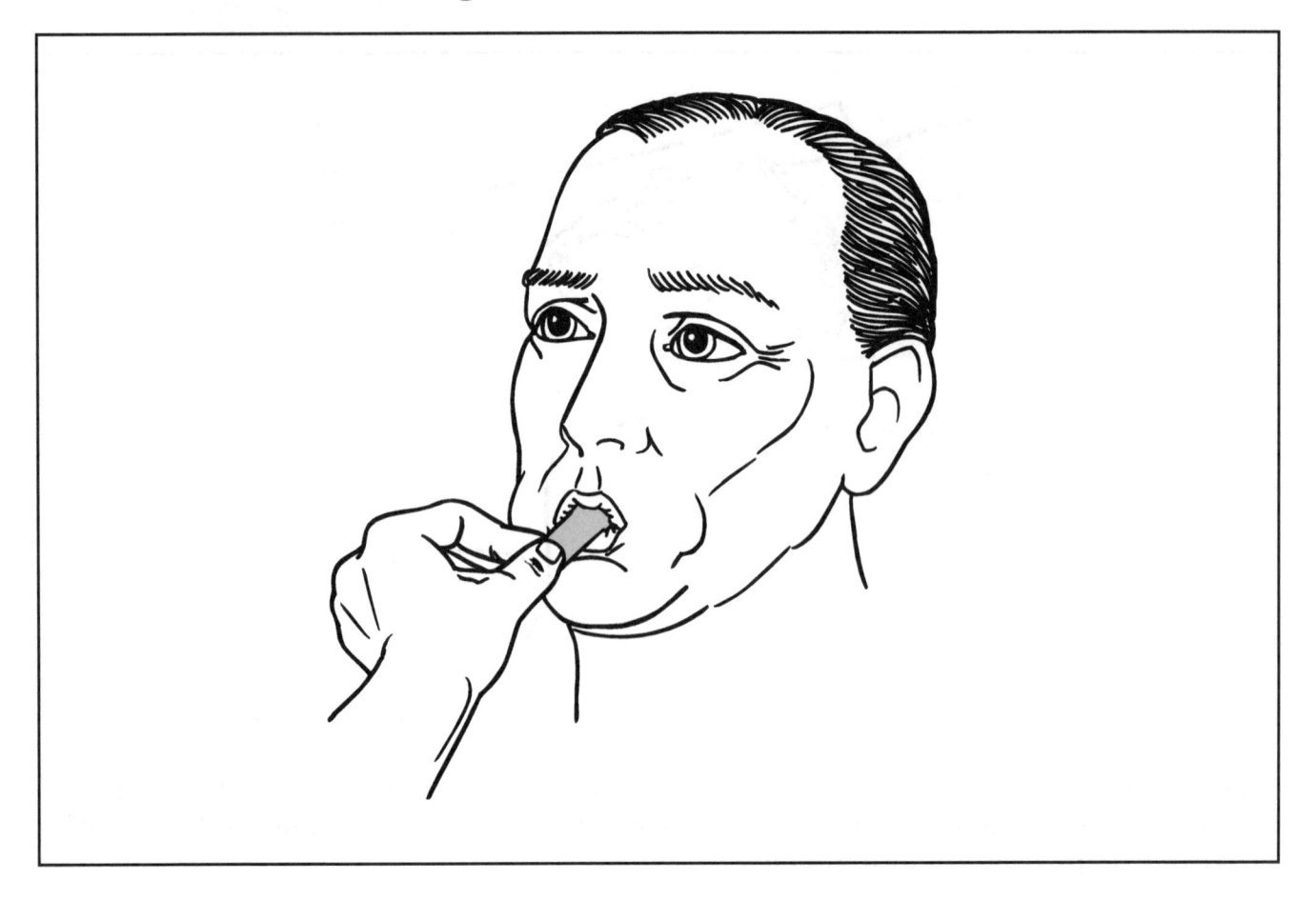

Chapter 8, continued

Put the top of the T of a Chewy Tube sideways in your mouth lengthwise (parallel with the earlobes) in front of your teeth. Do not bite down on it. Hold the long end securely and attempt to pull it out of your mouth. Use lip strength to keep the Chewy Tube in your mouth.

Release the outward pull on the tube and pull it back in using lip strength. Repeat 10 times as tolerated. Increase number of repetitions as tone increases.

Benefits

- assists in stretching and strengthening the inner cheeks
- assists in providing resistance for improved lip rounding
- improves lip seal

Squeezing and Kneading the Cheeks

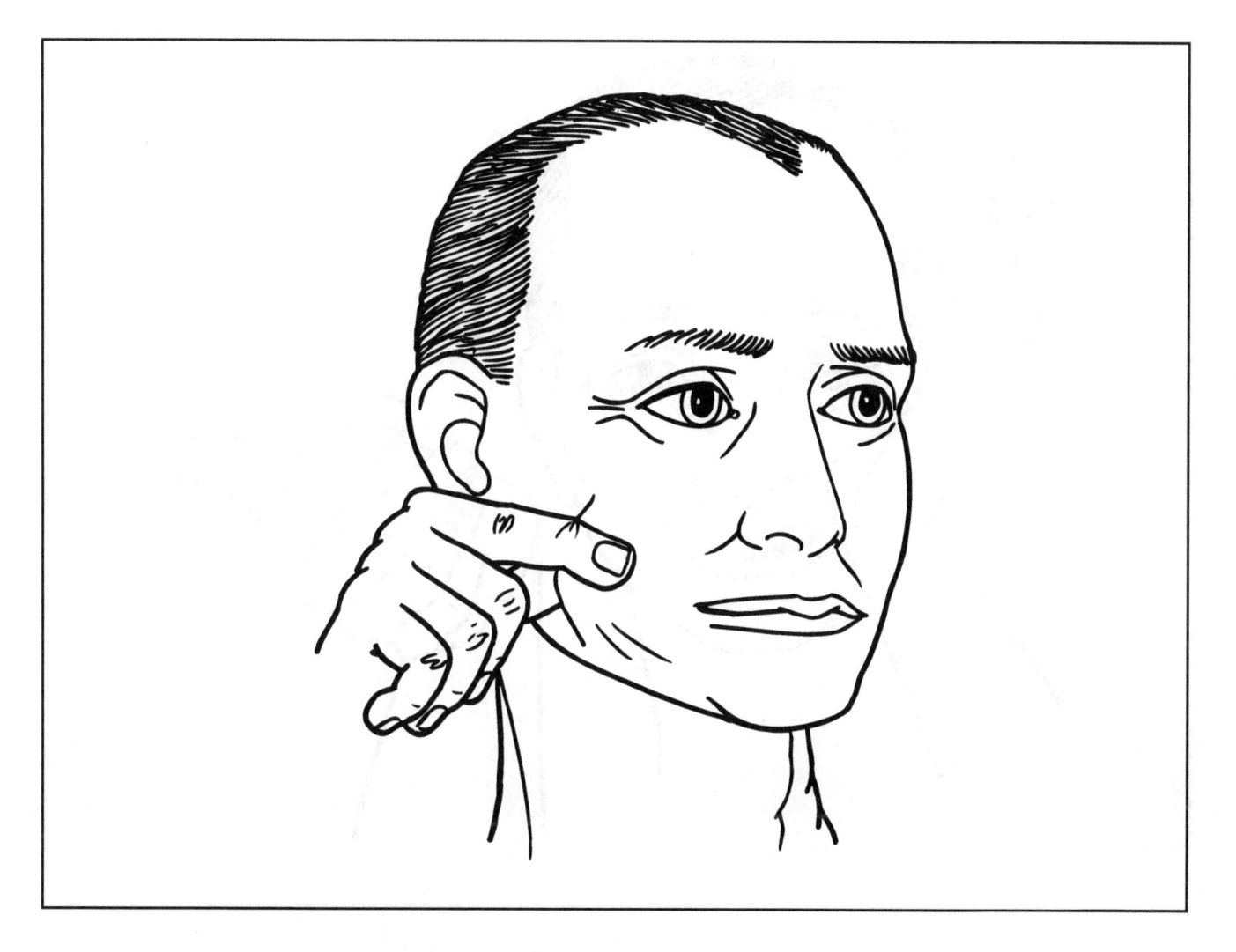

Chapter 8, continued

Grasp cheek in the middle with the index finger and thumb. Squeeze and knead the cheek, working to smooth out knotted musculature and/or to provide stimulation to weakened muscle tissue. Do each side one at a time or alternate from one side to the other using one hand on each cheek. Knead all the way around the cheeks, starting in the middle and moving in a circle.

Benefit

- smooths, stretches, tones, and stimulates cheek musculature

Rocking Palm Cheek Stretch

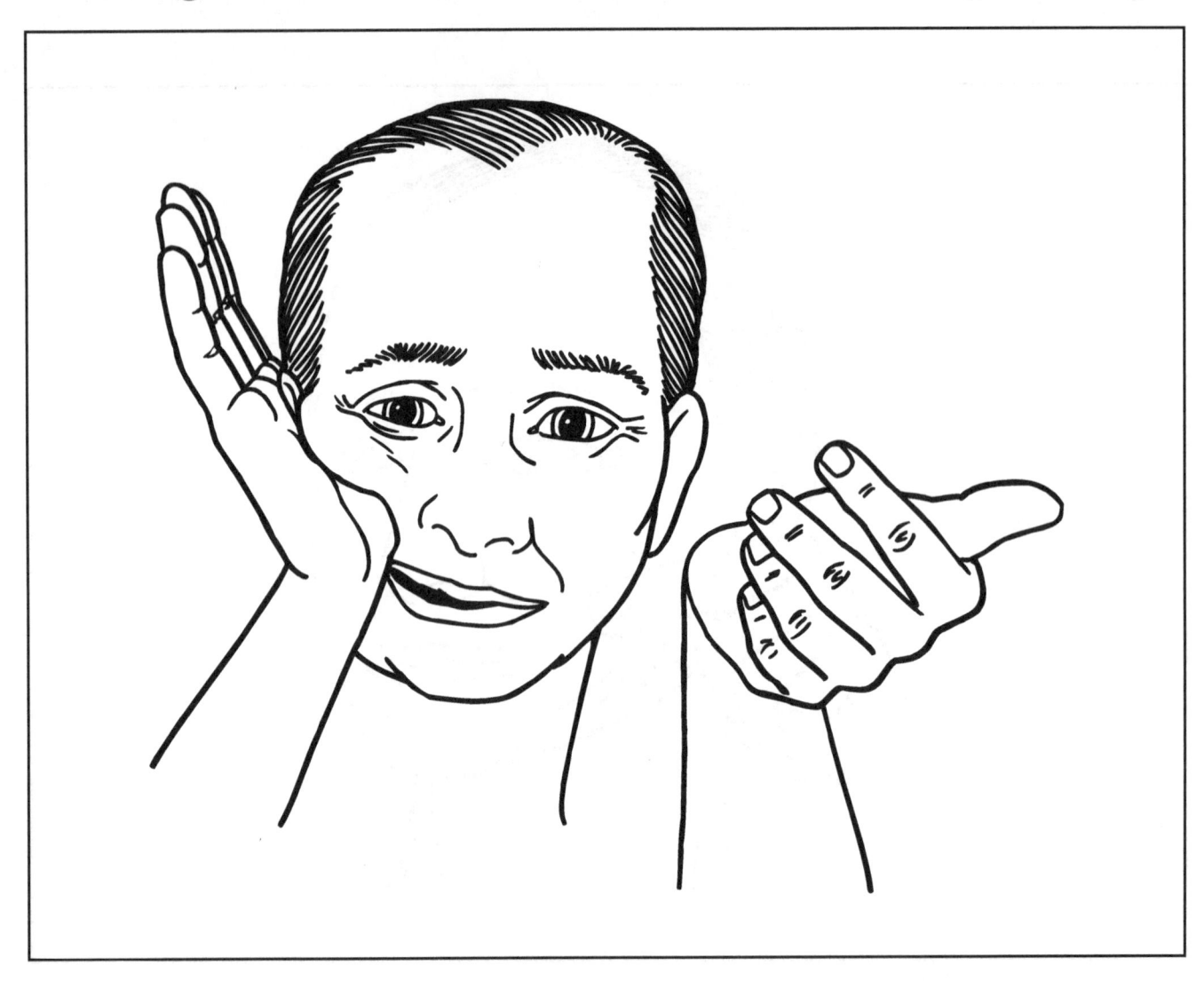

Chapter 8, continued

Put base of palm on cheekbone. Exert pressure on one cheek, pushing up and into cheekbone from the center. Switch to the other palm and cheekbone, exerting pressure for a count of 2. Rock back and forth from one cheek to the other. Lean elbows on the table for steady pressure and to assist in the rocking motion.

Benefit

- tones nasal area of cheeks

Buccal Cavity Pull

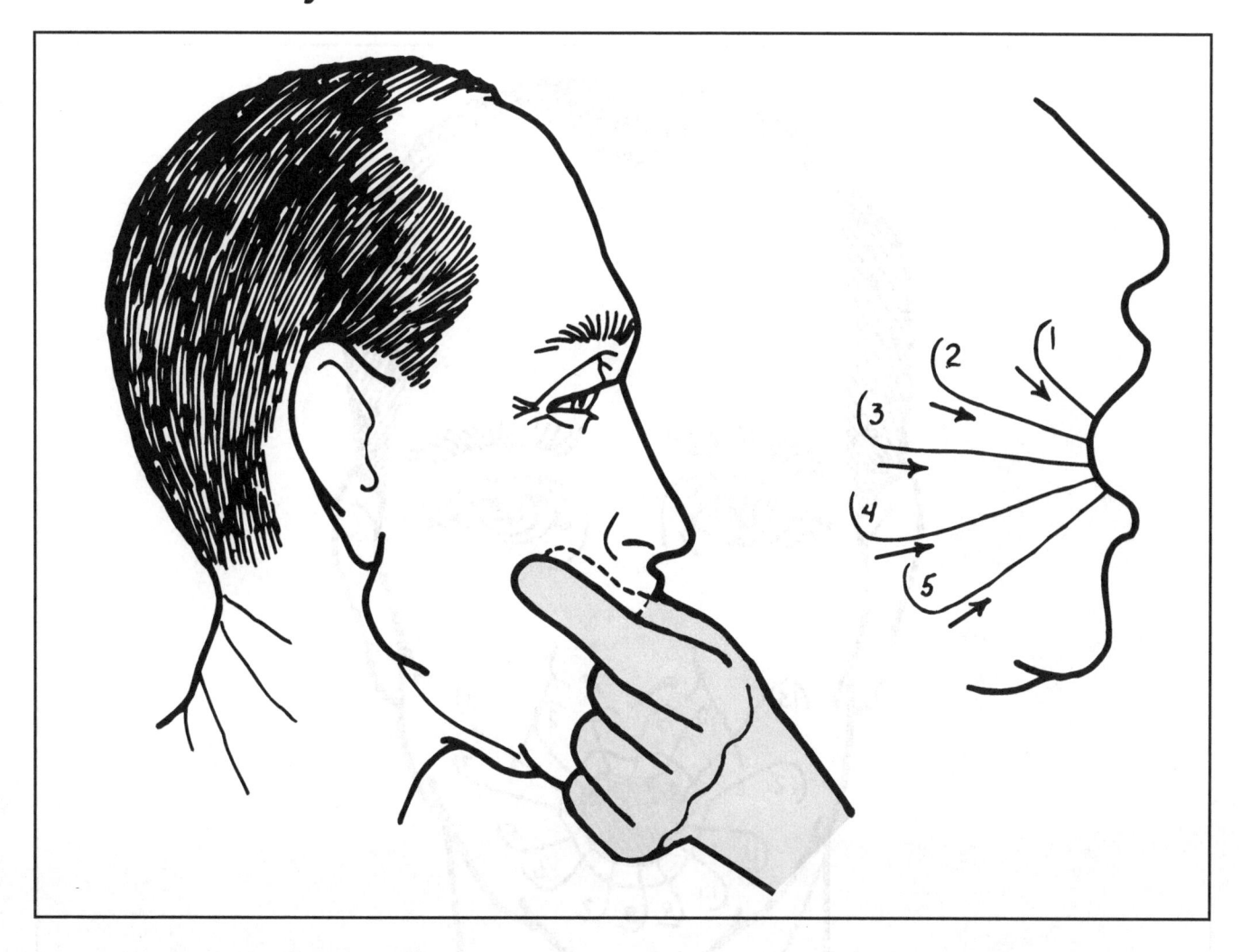

Chapter 8, continued

Put thumb inside mouth and index finger on outer cheek. Lightly squeeze index finger and thumb as you pull the cheek toward the corner of the lips. Follow the diagram for stretching cheeks. Go slowly to stretch restricted cheek musculature. Repeat. Perform exercise on the other cheek.

Benefits

○ encourages toning

○ stretches hypertonic or restricted cheek musculature

The Oral-Facial Therapy Exercise Book
2021 Edition

Extended Buccal Cavity Pull

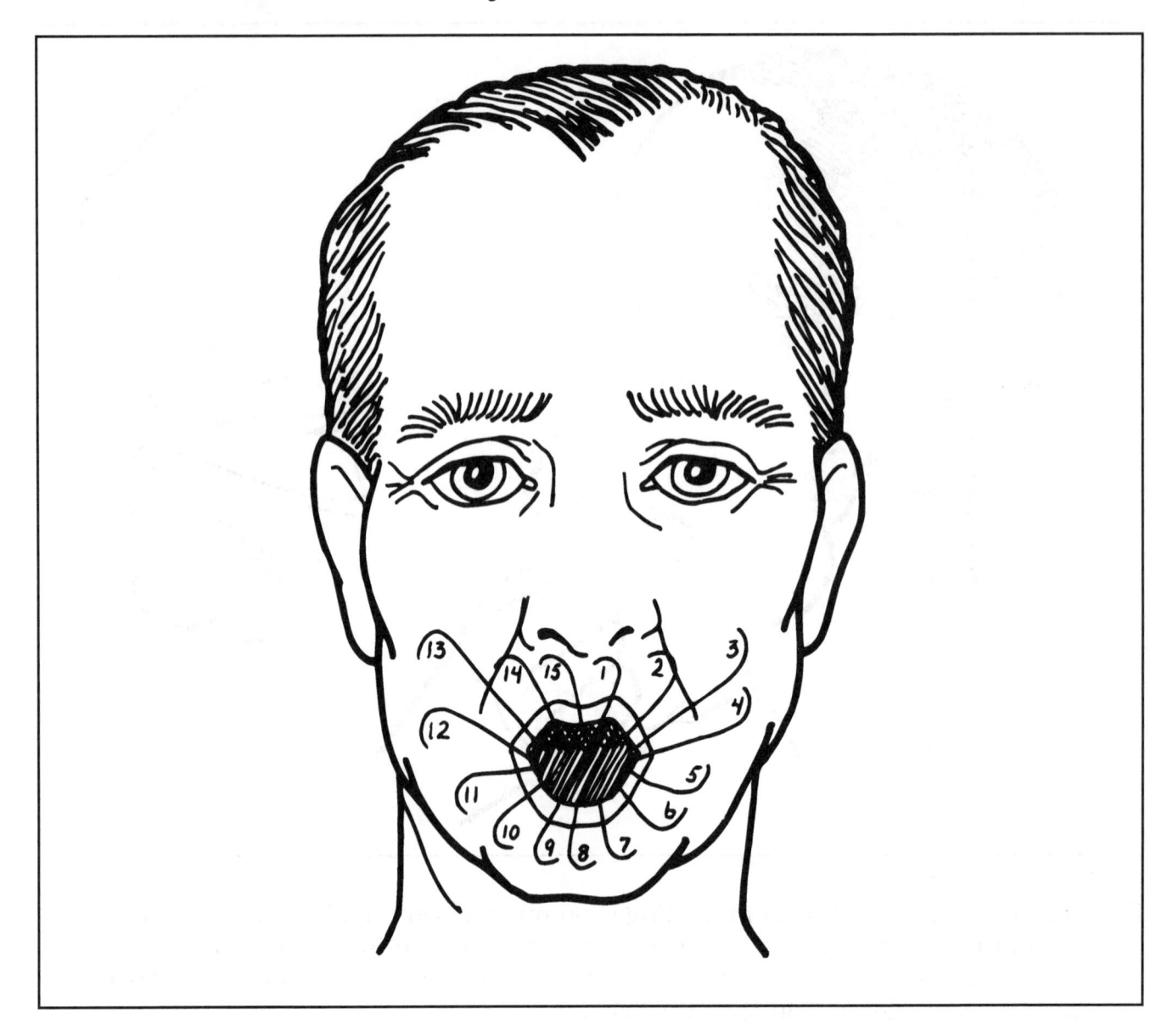

Chapter 8, continued

Put index finger inside mouth and thumb on outer cheek. Lightly squeeze index finger and thumb as you pull cheek toward lips. Move fingers and follow diagram to stretch cheeks. Stretch and pull sides evenly.

Benefit

- stretches and tones cheek musculature

Sustained Palm Massage of Cheeks

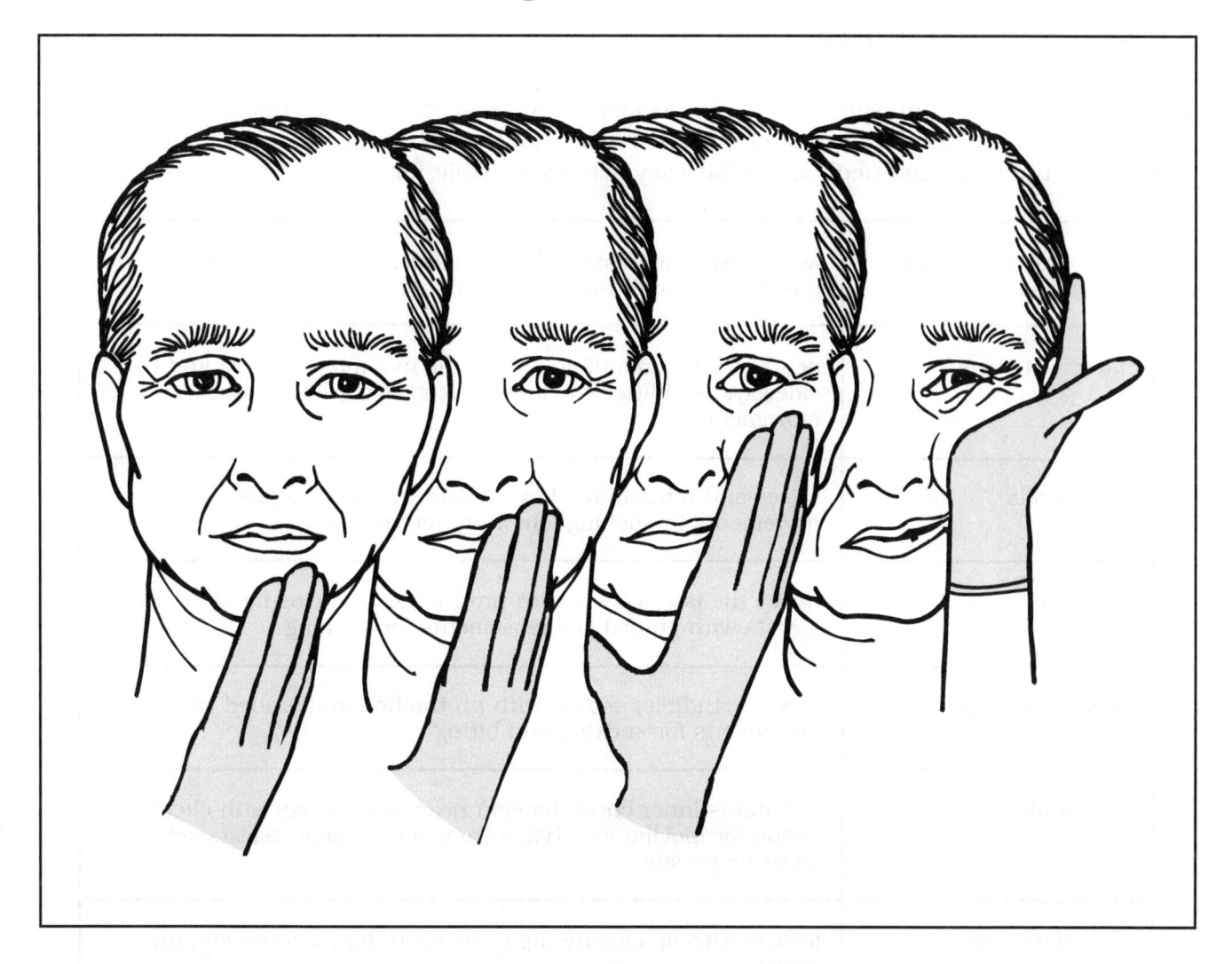

Chapter 8, continued

Place fingers from right hand on chin. Move fingers, then palm of hand from the chin over the right cheek to the end of the right eyebrow. Move upward only with sustained pressure, stretching the cheek musculature up and over the cheekbone. Continue pushing upward to the edge of the right eyebrow. Always start at the chin and push upward using smooth, even pressure. Repeat on the same side. Switch to left hand, continuously sliding upward to the left cheek, then following up to the edge of the left eyebrow. Repeat.

Benefit

- stretches and tones cheek musculature

Chapter 8, continued

Muscle Responsibility

There are a variety of muscle movements associated with speaking (e.g., opening the mouth for a cup, sucking on a straw, grinding food in the mouth). The following is a list of the muscles in the head and neck and what they are responsible for.

digastric, geniohyoid, myohyoid	assists with depressing the mandible; stabilizes the jaw; opening of mouth for spoon, cup, sucking, and munching
lateral pterygoid	depresses the mandible, draws the mandible forward and sideways, stabilizes the jaw, assists with graded jaw movements
temporalis	raises and retracts the jaw; assists with graded jaw movements in sucking, chewing, munching
masseter	raises the jaw, assists with protraction and closure of the jaw, assists with graded jaw movements for sucking
medial pterygoid	raises mandible; assists with protraction and graded jaw movements for sucking and biting
buccinator	maintains inner cheek tension near lips, assists with cheek action for moving food bolus from side-to-side, assists with lower lip tension
obicularis oris	assists with lip closure, lip protrusion, lip compression, lip elevation, lip tension
mentalis	wrinkles chin; assists with lower lip elevation, extended lip protrusion, and parting of the lips

All musculature assists in speech production. For specific sound per muscle production, see Table 1.5 of *Oral-Motor Assessment and Treatment: Ages and Stages* (Bahr 2001).

Chapter 9: Jaw Exercises

Temporomandibular Joint

The temporomandibular joint (TMJ) is a synovial joint that allows range of motion and relatively free movement between the bones that make up the joint. The movements of the muscle allow it to:

- depress
- elevate
- protrude
- retract
- lateralize
- rotate

The full range of motion allows for lip placement, tongue positioning, spatial configuration of the oropharynx, and laryngeal height.

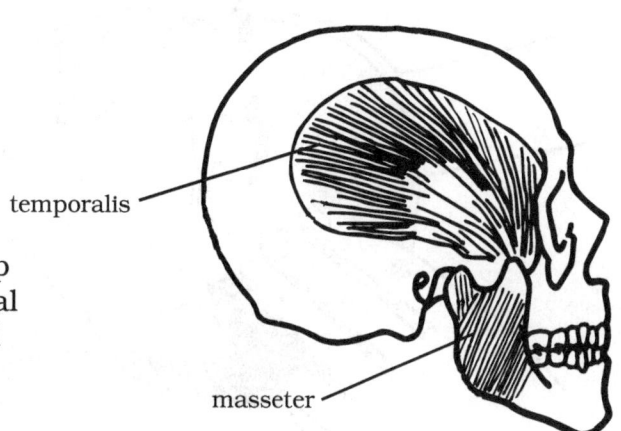

Lax or Hypo-functioning Joint

Lax joint ligaments can impair oral-motor function which causes errors in approximation and alignment. This is evidenced in individuals with Down syndrome. In individuals with cerebral palsy and traumatic brain injury, unilateral TMJ immobility is commonly experienced, causing asymmetry during oral-motor functioning. Errors in immobility (i.e., stiffness, lacking range of motion) are evidenced as drooling, difficulty chewing, difficulty munching with proper placement onto the molars, difficulty opening and closing the jaw in a hinge-like fashion, pocketing of food in the cheeks, biting on a cup or straw for stability, and loss of liquid when drinking with a cup.

Oral-motor massage and postural strategies will help create normal tone in the TMJ and surrounding areas. They will also help to strengthen tongue elevation, achieve lip closure, maintain jaw stability, and improve resonance and speech intelligibility as well as decrease drooling. Stop any interventions that may cause hyper- or high tone. Interventions that can increase tone are tapping, resistance, and icing.

Restricted, Stiff, or Hyper-functioning Joint

Massaging tense TMJ musculature can help reduce tone. Long, striated strokes are used to stretch and relax musculature. Warm compresses to the TMJ, stretches, yawns, breathwork, and communication strategies (e.g., positive messages, inquiry) are also effective in relieving restrictive musculature.

Chapter 9, *continued*

Temporalis Release

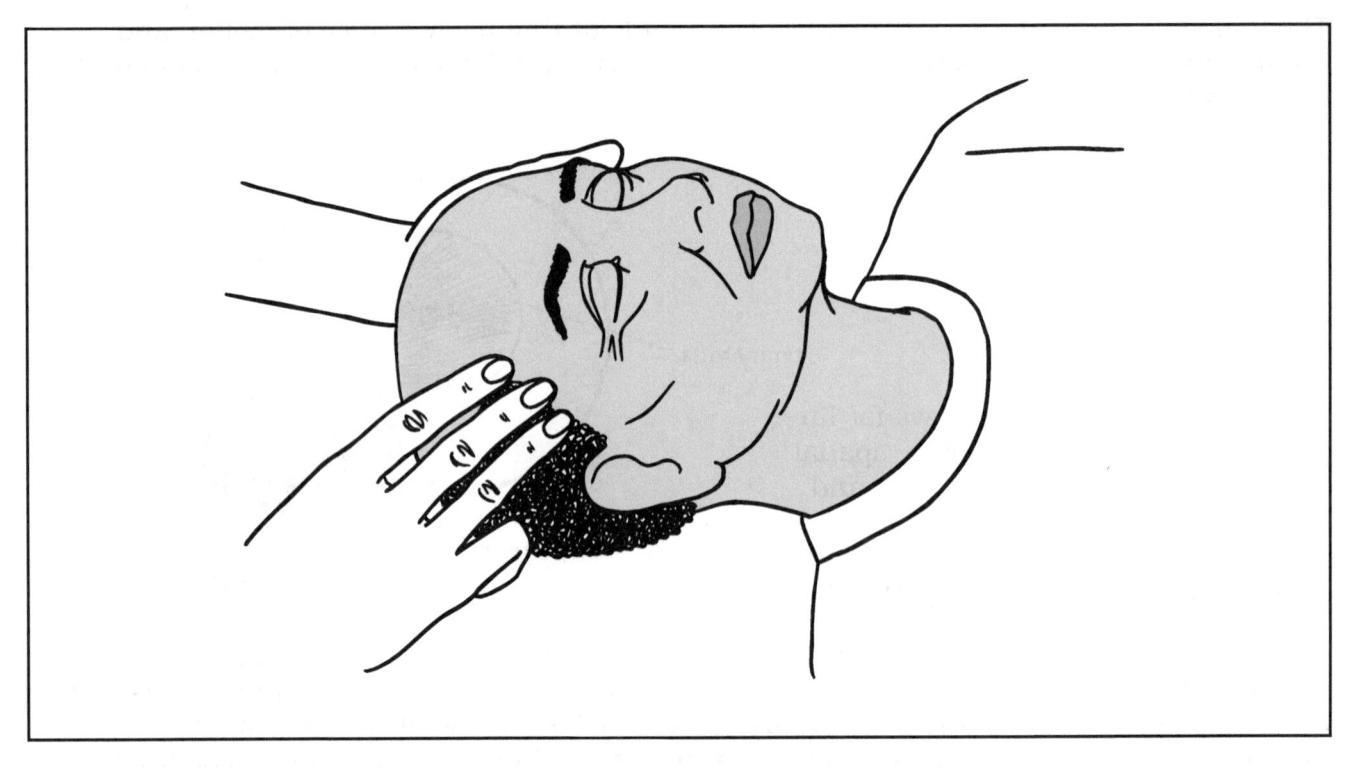

Press three fingers against the temporalis area on one side of the client's head at the level of the forehead. Move the scalp in small circles. If a painful spot is found, hold the pressure over it for five seconds. Move fingers to an adjacent spot and repeat, relieving bound musculature and stored tension as you go. Do both sides of the head simultaneously.

Encourage the individual to yawn or sigh during the exercise. Be open to discuss any emotional release or mental block that emerges as a result of freeing the musculature of the head. Ask the individual where the tension or pain has shifted. The client may respond "my shoulder," "my neck," "my nose," or "my leg." The ache may shift several times. Remind the individual that this is a process and over time, with practice, the imbalances, pains, and weakness will improve.

> Note: If you are unsure whether an intervention will help, try it. Our muscle and soft tissue system is so interconnected. Many times pain and muscle restriction, imbalance, or weakness is interdependent upon a group of muscles working together. Work the whole area. Ask for the individual's input. Body knowledge is amazing. Just ask the client to talk about his body. Where does he feel pain, sensitivity, restriction of movement?
>
> Be sure to note all findings and report them to the client's primary physician. A referral to physical, occupational, or massage therapy may be indicated.

Chapter 9, *continued*

Stabilizing the Jaw

Stabilizing the jaw allows freedom of fine motor movement of the tongue and facial musculature. It is important to stabilize the jaw when seeking to isolate a particular facial or tongue movement for controlled graded movement of the muscle.

Bite Blocks

A bite block is used to:

- stabilize and maintain the client's jaw in desired positions to strengthen and increase range of motion of the tongue

- allow access to the oral cavity when working with clients who exhibit a strong bite reflex

- increase range of motion of jaw through gradually increased bite block sizes

- strengthen the client's jaw by having him bite down on the bite block

For hygienic purposes, clients should have their own bite block apparatus. Clean the apparatus with soap and hot water before and after each session. Items that may be used as bite blocks or jaw stabilizers are:

- tongue depressor

- Chewy Tube

- end of toothbrush

- corks – varying sizes of corks make effective bite and resistance blocks (Put gauze around the cork or a finger cot over the cork to make it easier to hold onto, for hygienic purposes, and to contain pieces of the cork if it crumbles.)

- rolled gauze

When to use a bite block:

1. To gradually increase the client's jaw opening, begin with a narrow item such as a Chewy Tube, a tongue depressor, or the end of a toothbrush. Before and after this exercise, have the client open his mouth as wide as possible to establish a baseline and to gauge improvement. Note muscle resistance to each item as you place slightly larger bite blocks in the client's mouth. Repeat from smallest to largest bite block, again noting the resistance of the jaw.

Chapter 9, continued

2. To stabilize the client's jaw for the tongue exercises, place the bite block between the upper and lower central incisors. Instruct the client not to bite down on the block, but to relax her teeth on the block. Perform the tongue exercises with intermittent breaks to rest the jaw musculature.

   Have the client attempt to perform the tongue strengthening exercises using various sizes of bite blocks. Practice subsequent tongue range and strength abilities with and without the bite block.

3. If a bite reflex is probable, roll gauze into a cylinder of desired thickness and use it as a bite block. A bite reflex is common in infants and children.

Head and Jaw Stability

If the client lacks tongue mobility, he might overcompensate by using his jaw. His tongue may be flaccid or move very little so he compensates by using his jaw to raise and lower it. By stabilizing the client's jaw, you will be able to clearly assess the client's tongue strength and range of motion more accurately. The following suggestions will help you stabilize the client's jaw.

To stabilize the client's head and jaw:

- Grasp the back of the client's head with your index finger and thumb at the base of the neck as it joins the skull, approximately two inches behind the ears. Once the client's head is propped into place, use your other hand to stabilize the jaw as described above. You may wish to use an assistant to aid in stabilizing the client's head.

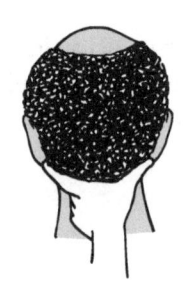

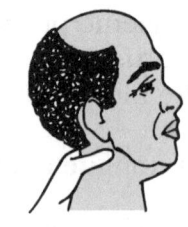

- Depress the client's lower lip with your index finger. Then depress his jaw with your middle finger, holding his mouth open varying degrees according to tongue tip stretch desired.

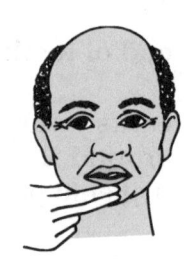

- Place your thumb under the client's chin to grip the jaw and further stabilize it. This allows independent movement of the raising, retracting, lateralizing, or protrusion of the tongue.

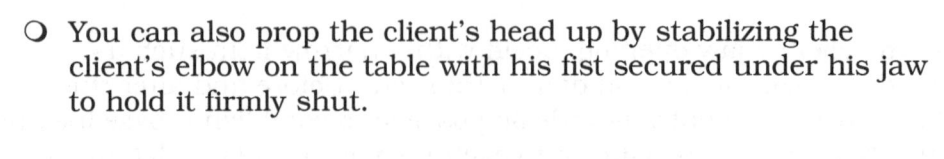

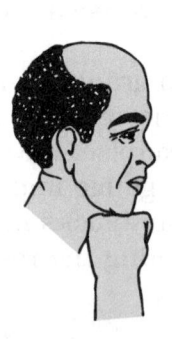

- You can also prop the client's head up by stabilizing the client's elbow on the table with his fist secured under his jaw to hold it firmly shut.

The Oral-Facial Therapy Exercise Book
2021 Edition

Releasing Jaw Tension

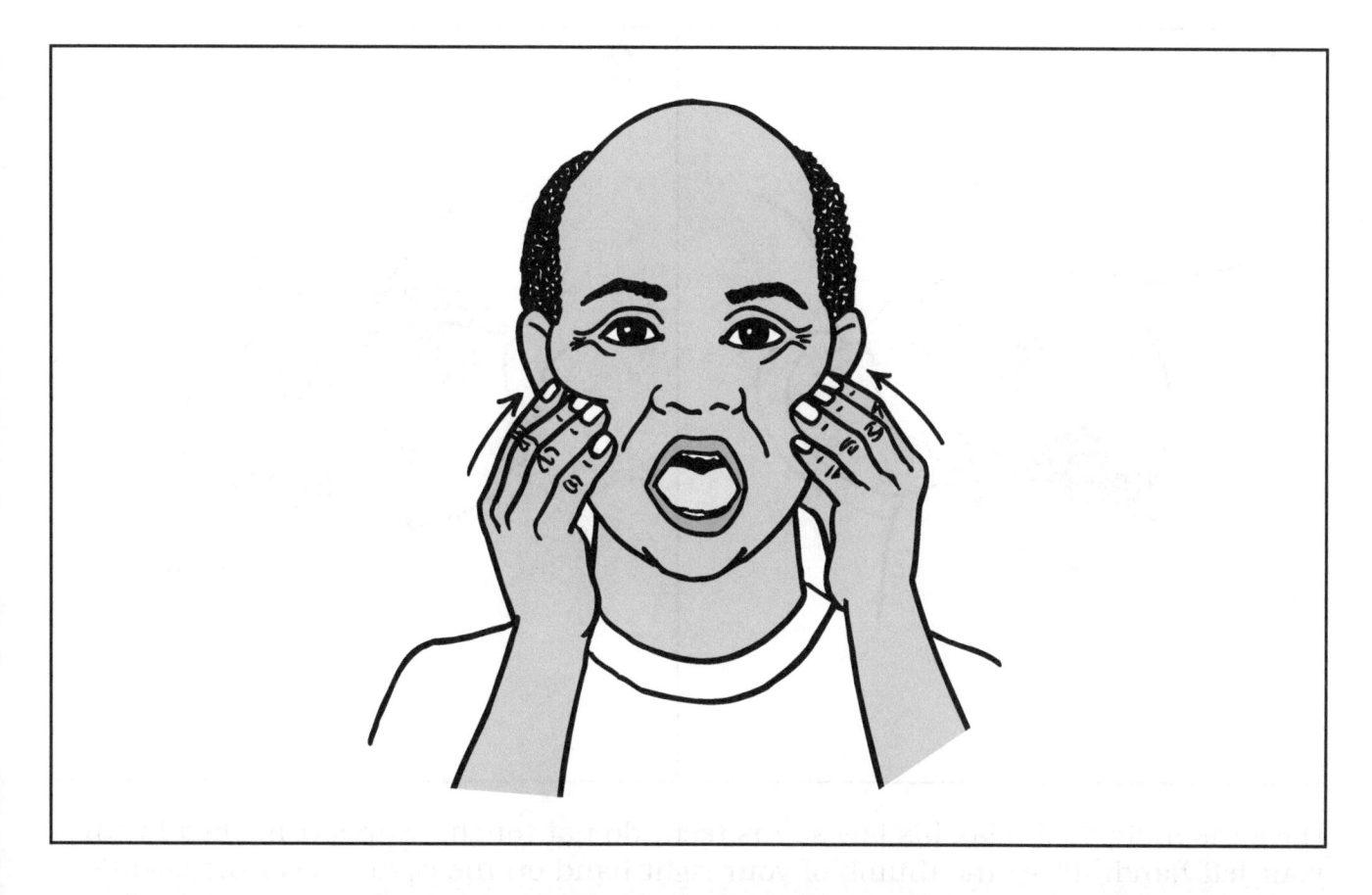

Chapter 9, *continued*

Place the fingertips of both hands on your upper jaw. Press firmly and slowly with equal pressure on both sides, letting your fingers go through the surface tissue of the cheeks until you feel the resistance of the muscle that runs from the cheek to the lower jaw.

You may feel the resistance as hardness or soreness. Increase pressure until you begin to feel discomfort. Breathe deeply to release any tension in the jaw. Open and close the jaw, sounding "AH" loudly to release tension. Continue to apply on and off pressure for 30 seconds. Repeat once as tolerated.

Benefits

○ releases tension

○ reduces difficulties with overall head and neck pain

Jaw Massage

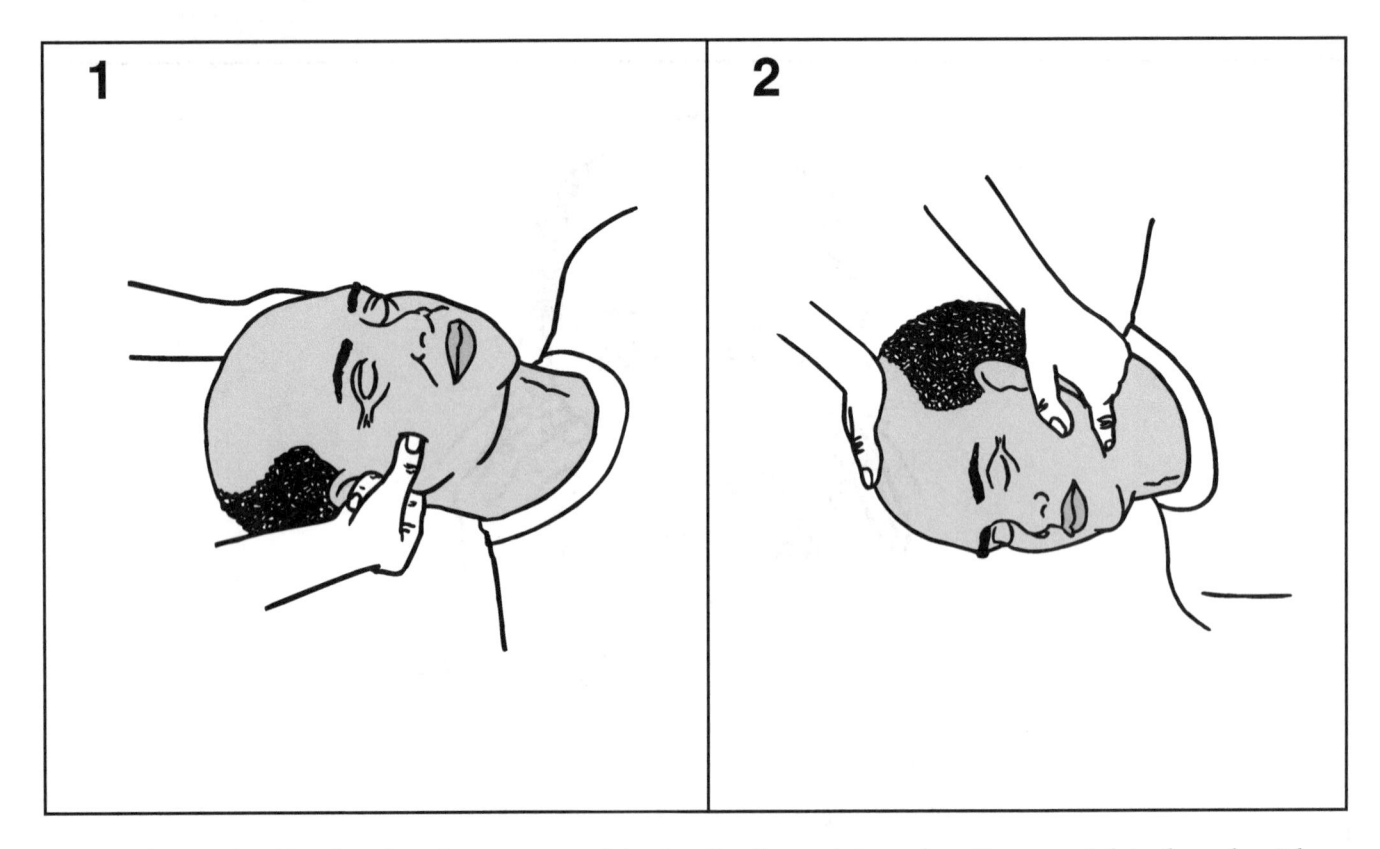

Chapter 9, *continued*

1

2

Have the individual relax his jaw so his teeth do not touch. Support his head with your left hand. Place the thumb of your right hand on the right side of the client's head where his jaw meets his TMJ as shown in picture 1. Apply pressure slowly and gently. The client should not be wincing or clenching his jaw. Make circular motions with the thumb before releasing.

Move a half of an inch down toward the tip of the jaw and repeat. To secure thumb pressure, place a stabilizing finger or two below the jaw as shown in picture 2. To stretch these muscles, have the individual open his mouth. Repeat on the other side in the same manner.

> Note: Releasing and toning this musculature is a process. Healing takes place over time. It may be necessary to request other intervention strategies such as neuromuscular massage therapy, physical therapy, or occupational therapy to further assist the rehabilitation process.

Benefit

- releases jaw and neck tension

Stretch and Massage

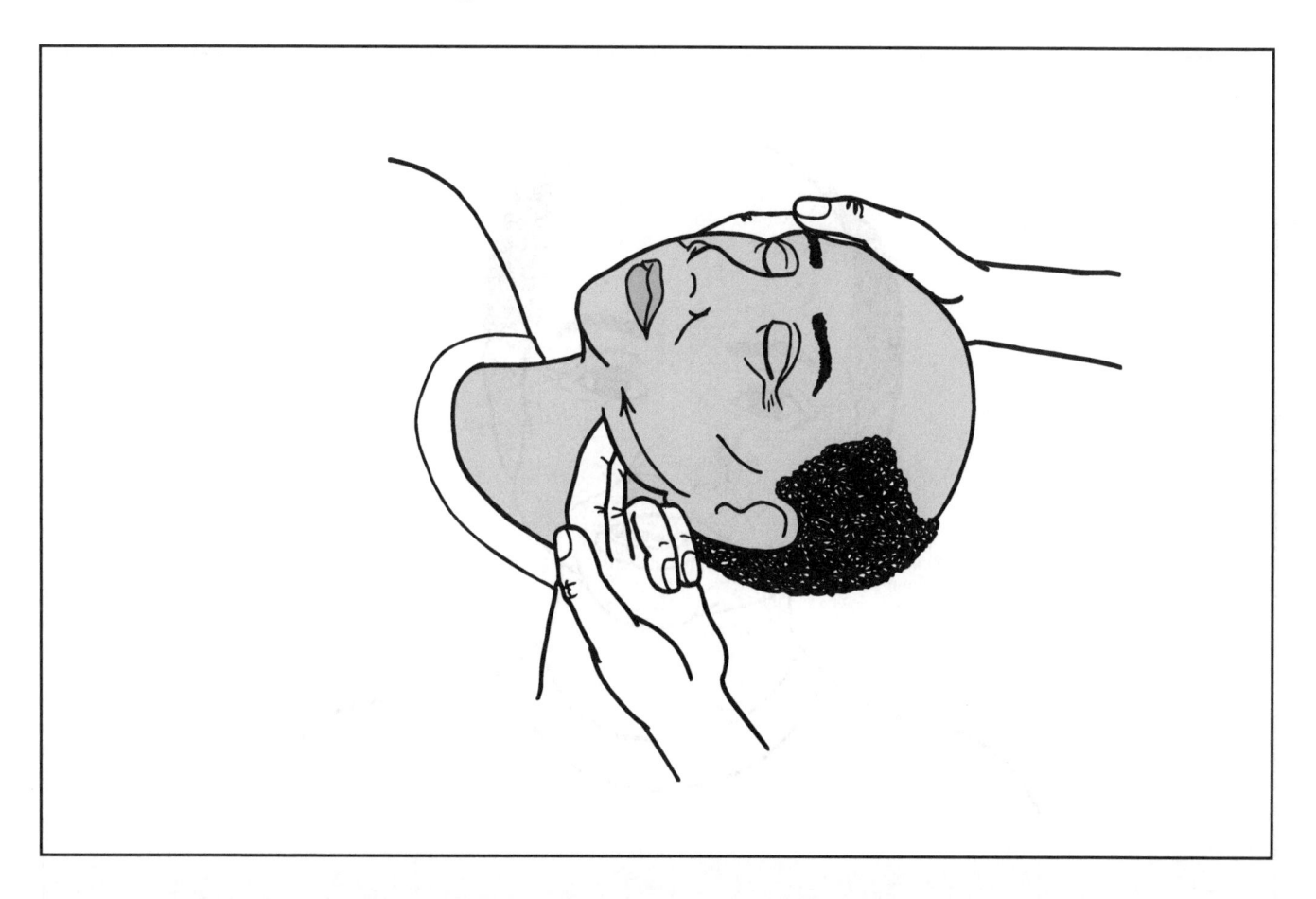

Chapter 9, continued

Gently support the client's head with one hand. Place your other hand under the client's jaw by his earlobe. Apply pressure with your fingertips as you move in half-inch increments along the length of the jaw to the point of the chin.

Remember, this is a sensitive area where many muscle groups come together so it can be tender. Your application of pressure can send waves of relief to the temporalis muscle, the neck, the tongue, and the face.

> Note: The client may want to apply the pressure himself. Remind him to go slowly.

Benefit

○ massages underneath tongue, releasing jaw tension

Jaw Rotation

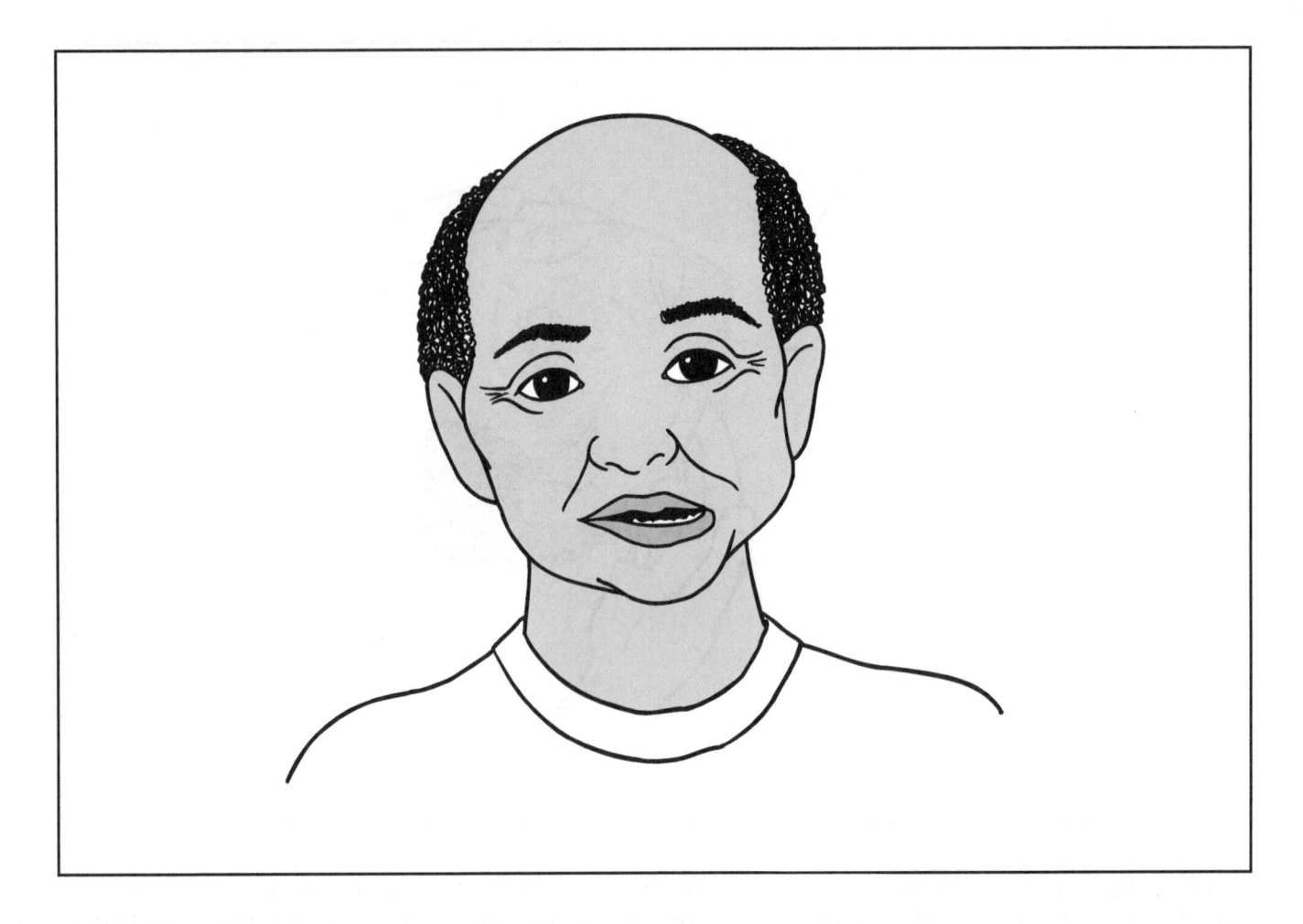

Chapter 9, continued

Move the jaw in a circular pattern. Begin with a small mouth opening and move it clockwise 3 times. Then move it counter-clockwise 3 times. Increase to a wider mouth opening and move the jaw clockwise and counter-clockwise 3 times each. Repeat 3 times as tolerated. You may wish to massage the masseter muscle before and after this exercise.

Benefit

- stretches and strengthens range of motion for chewing and munching

Jaw Opening Resistance

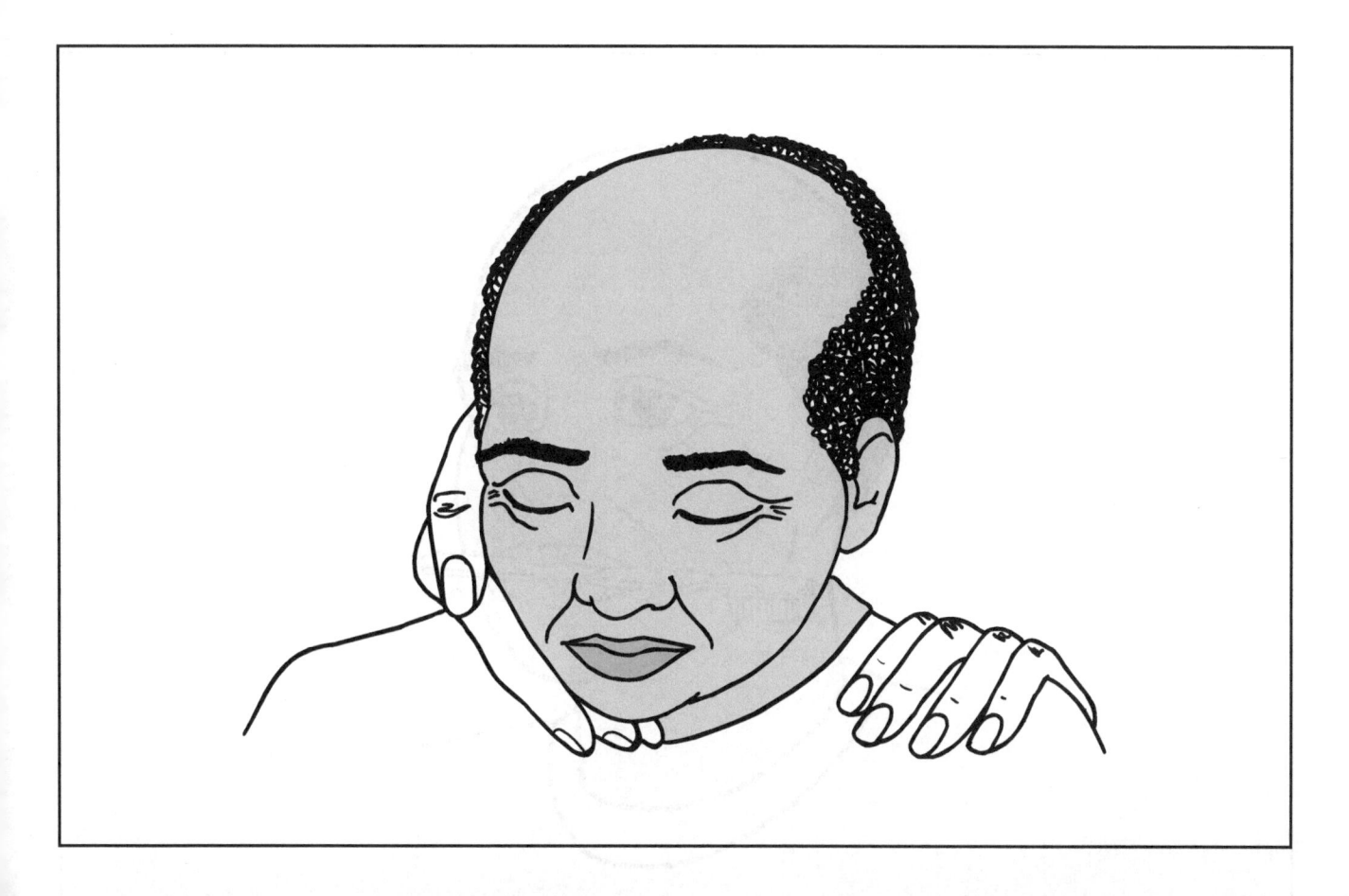

Chapter 9, *continued*

Position the client's head so that it is secure and upright. (If the individual is lying on a bed, hold the top of his head with one hand). Stand behind the client and place your hand gently on the bottom of his chin. Have the client try to open his jaw while you apply light resistance. Then allow the jaw to open fully. Repeat 2 to 3 times. Remind the client to relax his neck.

As jaw strength and range of motion increases, offer slightly more resistance. Again remind the individual to relax the neck.

Benefit

- strengthens the jaw for opening and downward motion

Decrease Jaw Clench

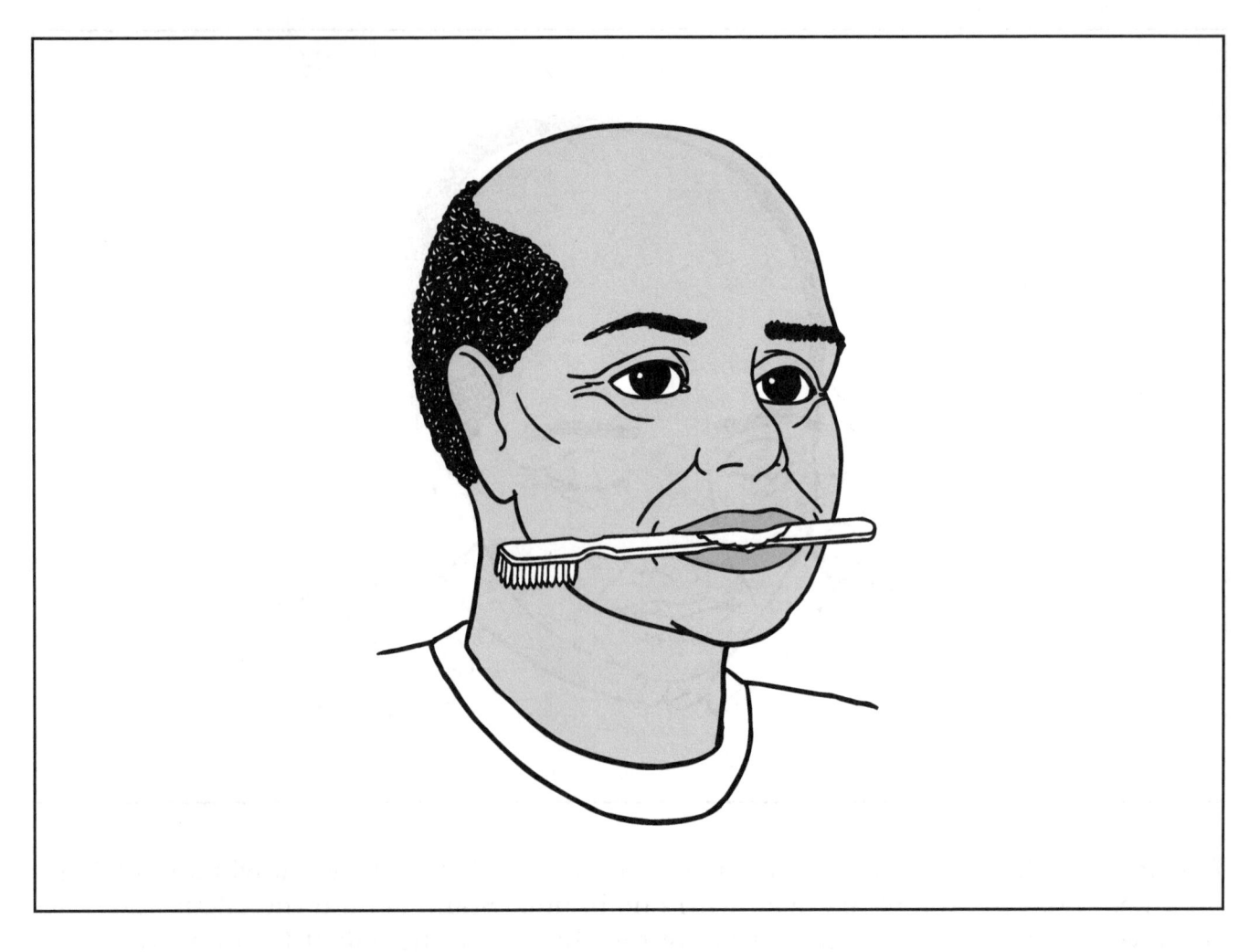

Chapter 9, *continued*

Place a toothbrush horizontally in the mouth, directly behind the front teeth. Clench the toothbrush lightly for about 5 minutes. Repeat this exercise several times during the day.

Benefits

- reduces jaw pain, jaw clenching, and grinding of the teeth

- effective in reducing tinnitus (can occur as a result of excessive temporo-mandibular tension)

Chin Massage

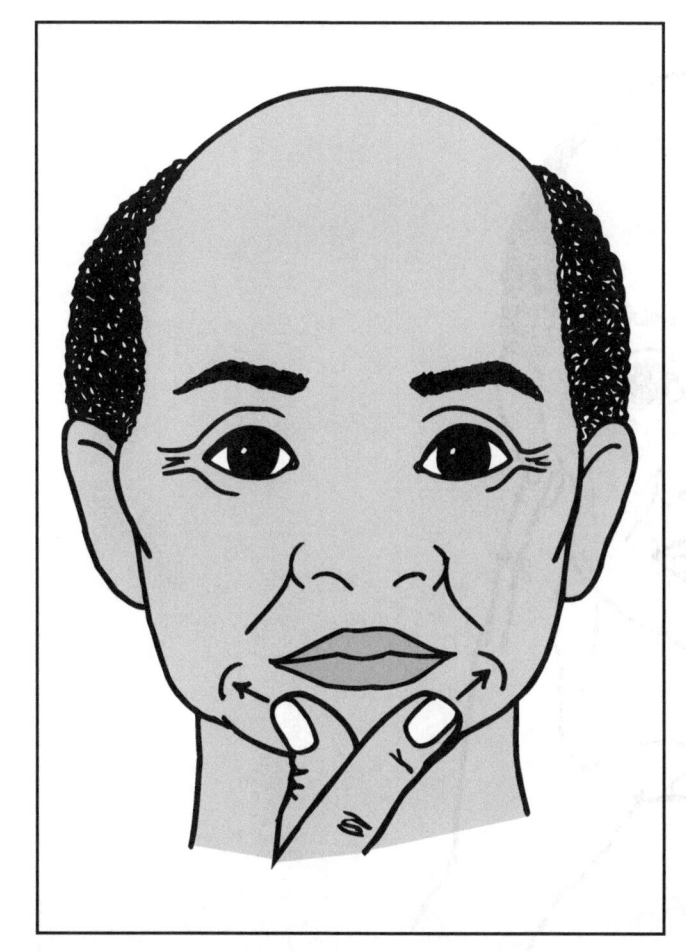

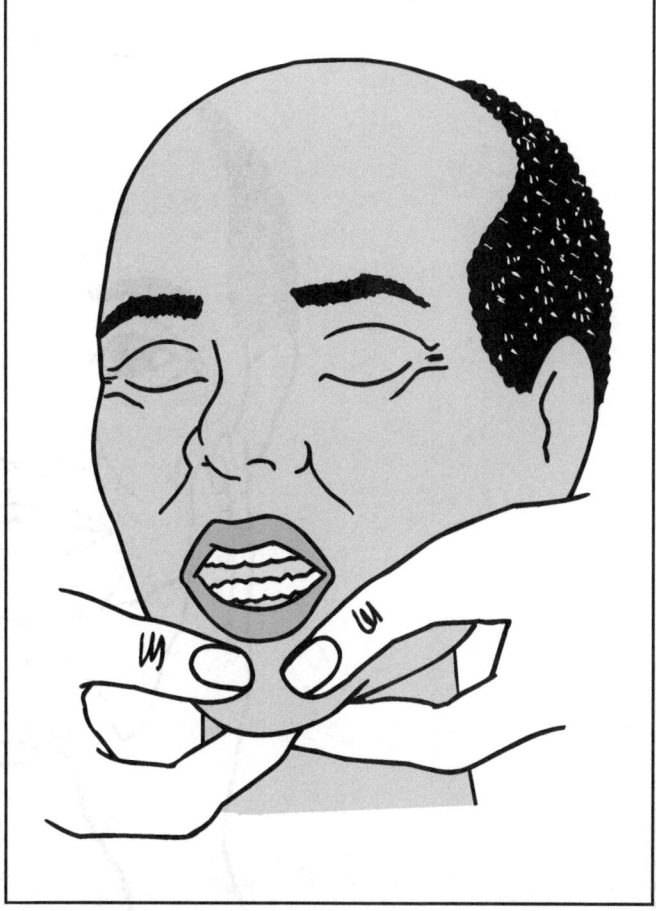

Chapter 9, continued

Rest index finger and thumb on the chin. Massage outward along the jaw line halfway up the cheek (toward the mandibular joint). Always start at the chin and massage up and outward only.

Massage the chin to reduce hypertonicity. Conversely, gently tap the chin to increase tone. If there is paralysis on one side, tap on that side and massage the unaffected side. In addition, massaging both sides will help build tone on the weakened side as well as stretch and relax the unaffected side.

Benefits

- reduces excessive or inappropriate tension
- improves muscle tone

Jaw Muscle Massage

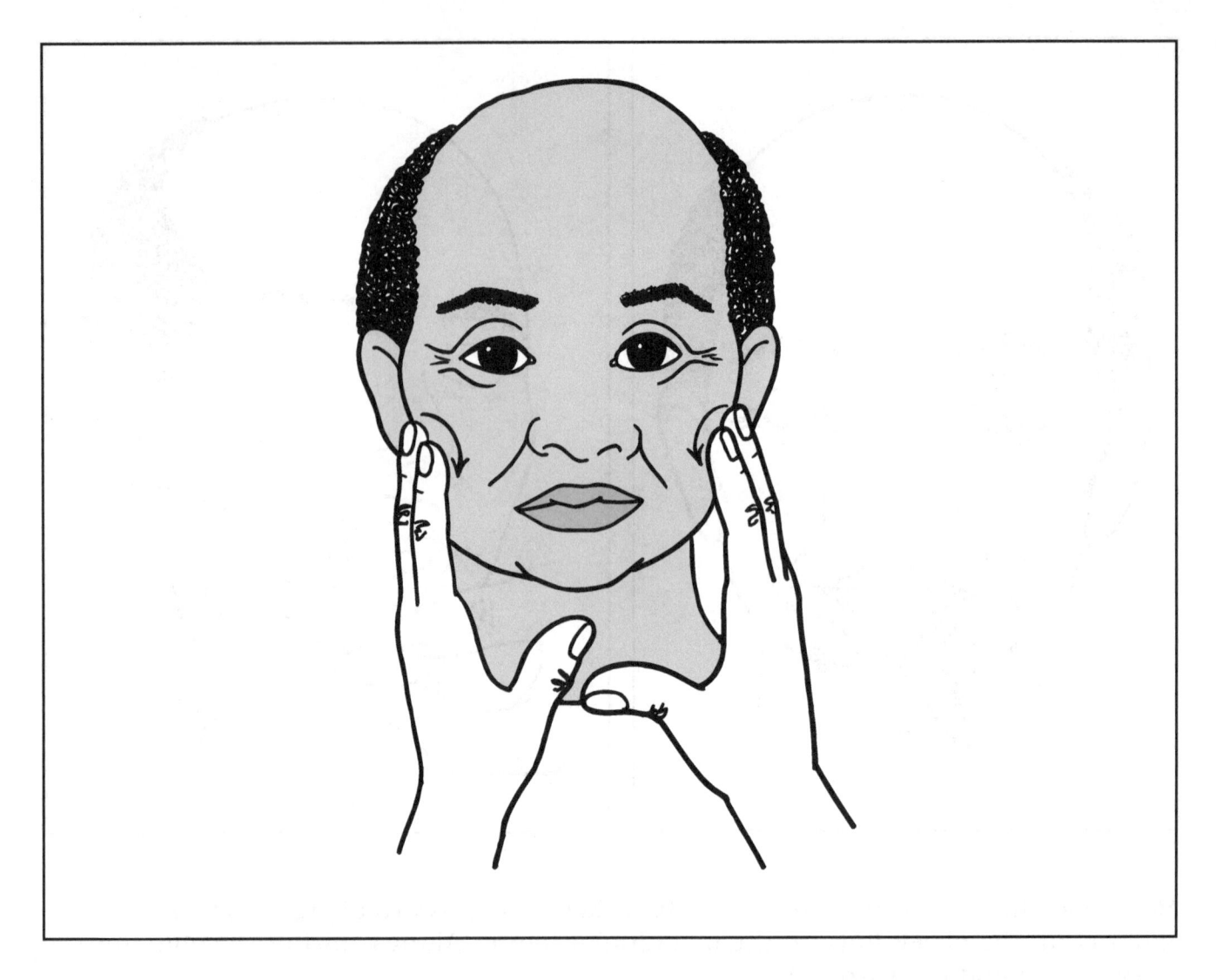

Chapter 9, continued

Apply gentle pressure with the index and middle fingers to temporomandibular joint on each side. Rub in a circular motion for 30 seconds. Keep jaw relaxed.

Benefits

- reduces jaw tightness and strain

- relaxes tight jaw muscles

- firms weak jaw muscles

Temple Massage

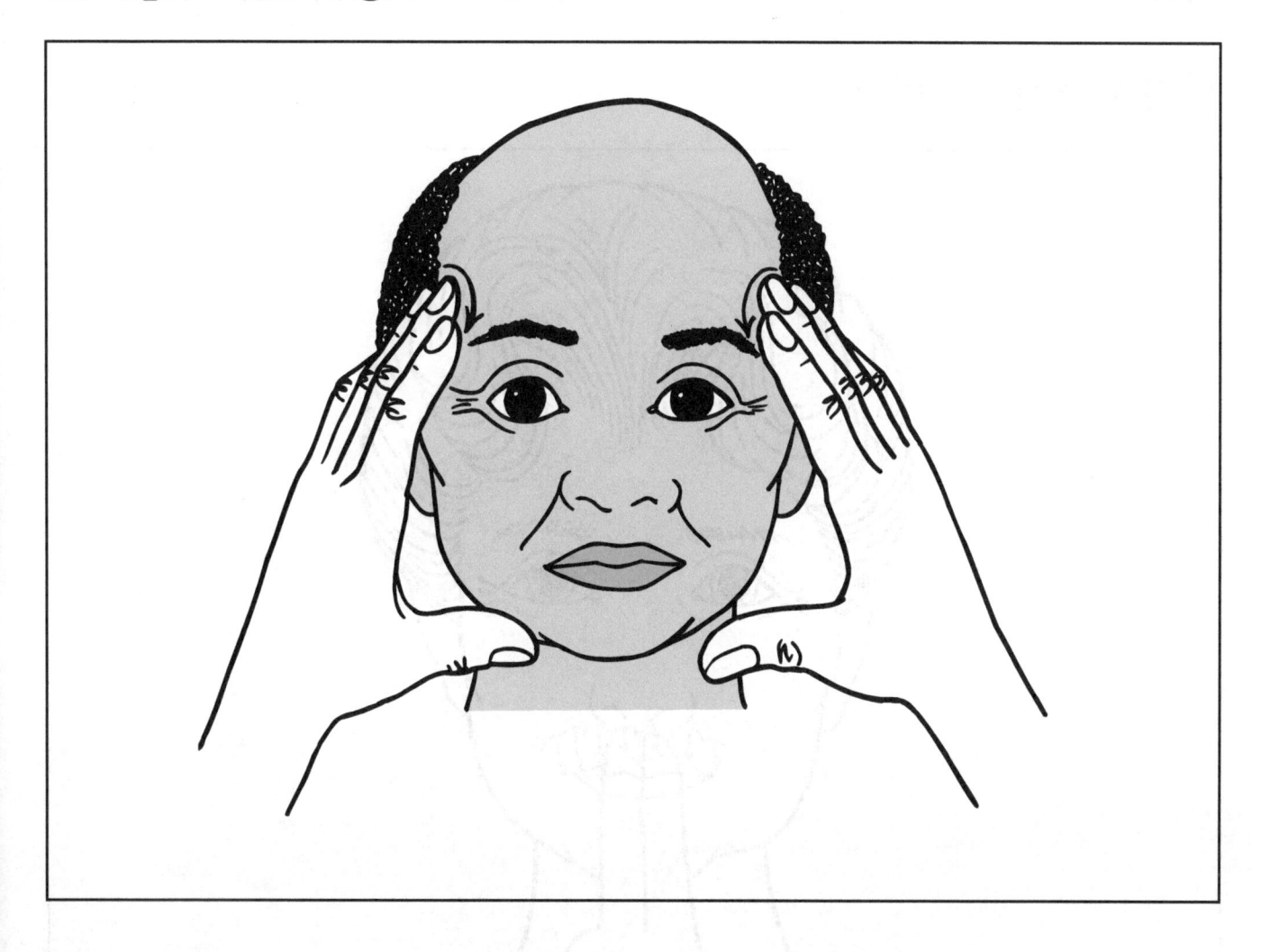

Chapter 9, continued

Place fingers on temples, applying light pressure. Rub in a circular motion. Maintain steady pressure to temple. Rest. Reverse circular motion.

Benefits

- relaxes temporomandibular joint

- reduces grimacing and facial strain

The Oral-Facial Therapy Exercise Book
2021 Edition

Chapter 10: Lip Exercises

Upper Lip Stretch

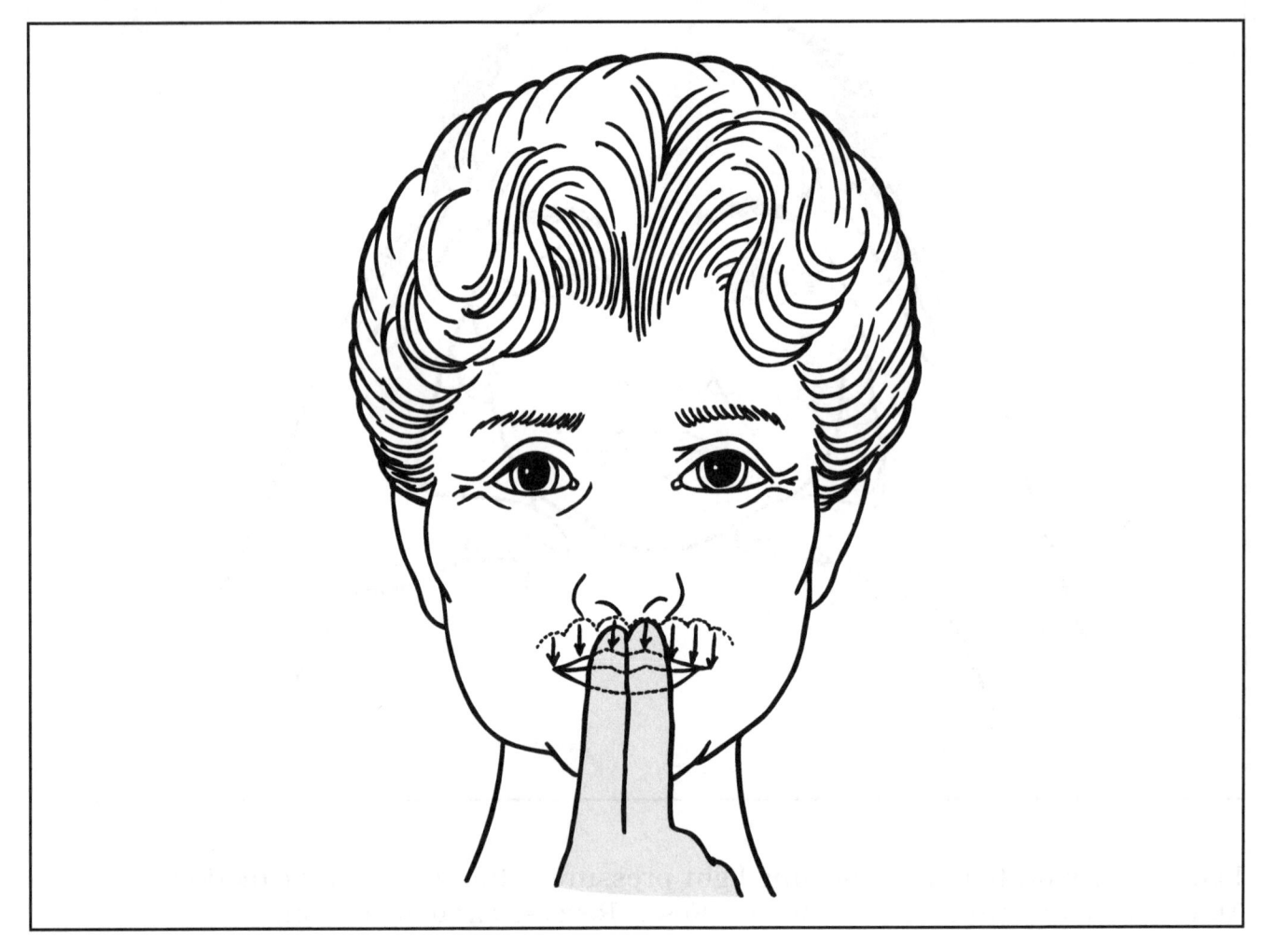

Begin with two fingers as shown at base of nose. Apply light pressure with downward motion. Repeat until you reach the corner of each sides of the upper lip. Go back to midline at nostrils and repeat on left side. Repeat 3 to 5 times on each side in slow, even, downward motions.

Benefits

- stretches and elongates upper lip
- approximates upper lip to lower lip
- improves lip closure

Corner of Upper Lip Downward Stretch   Chapter 10, *continued*

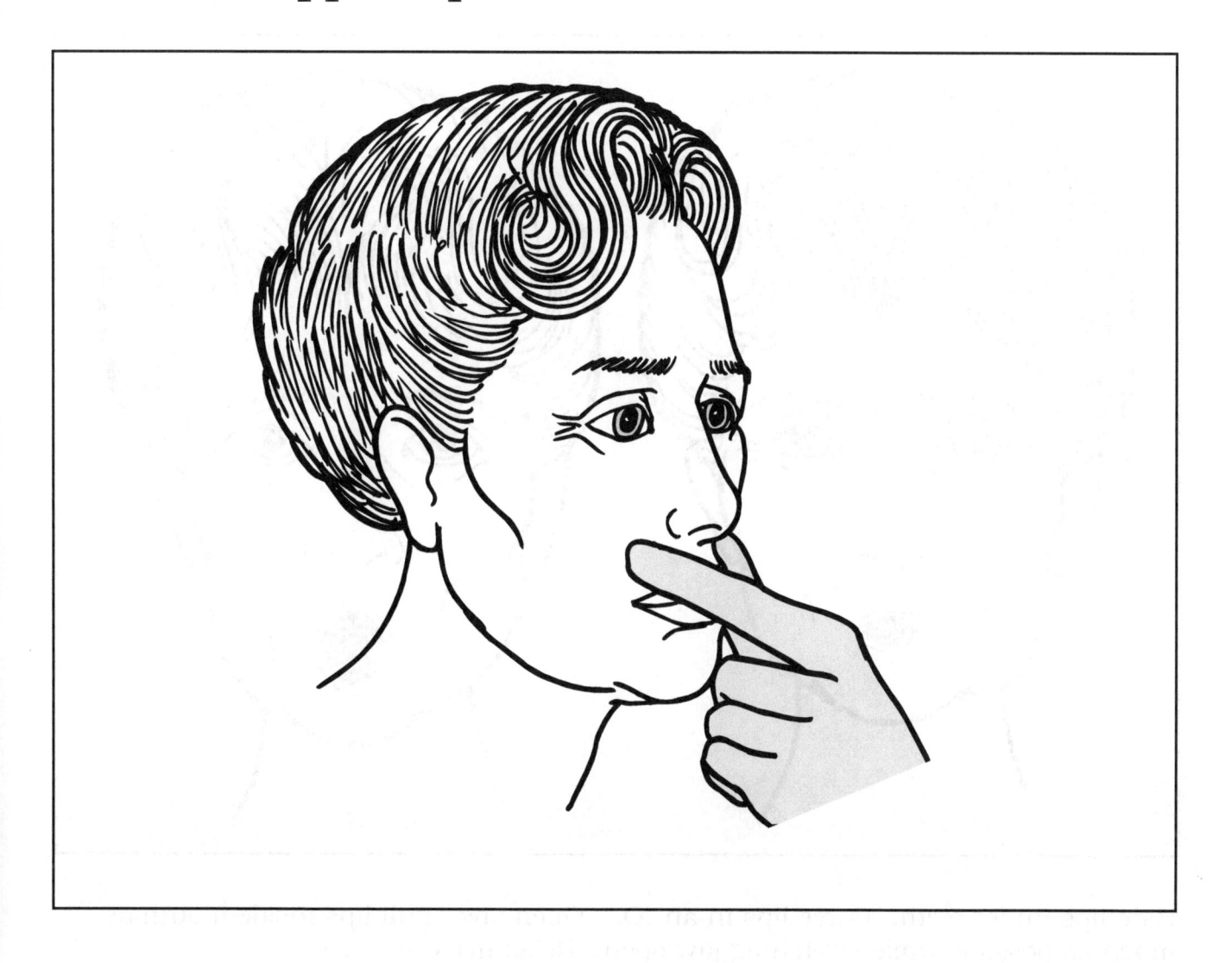

Place index finger on the corner of each side of the upper lip below the cheek. Place thumb on the other side of the upper lip. Apply pressure and press down for 30 seconds. Repeat 5 to 10 times.

Benefits

- stretches and elongates upper lip to form a seal for /p, b, m/ and to suck on a straw

- strengthens lip closure to reduce drooling

"O" Exercise

Chapter 10, continued

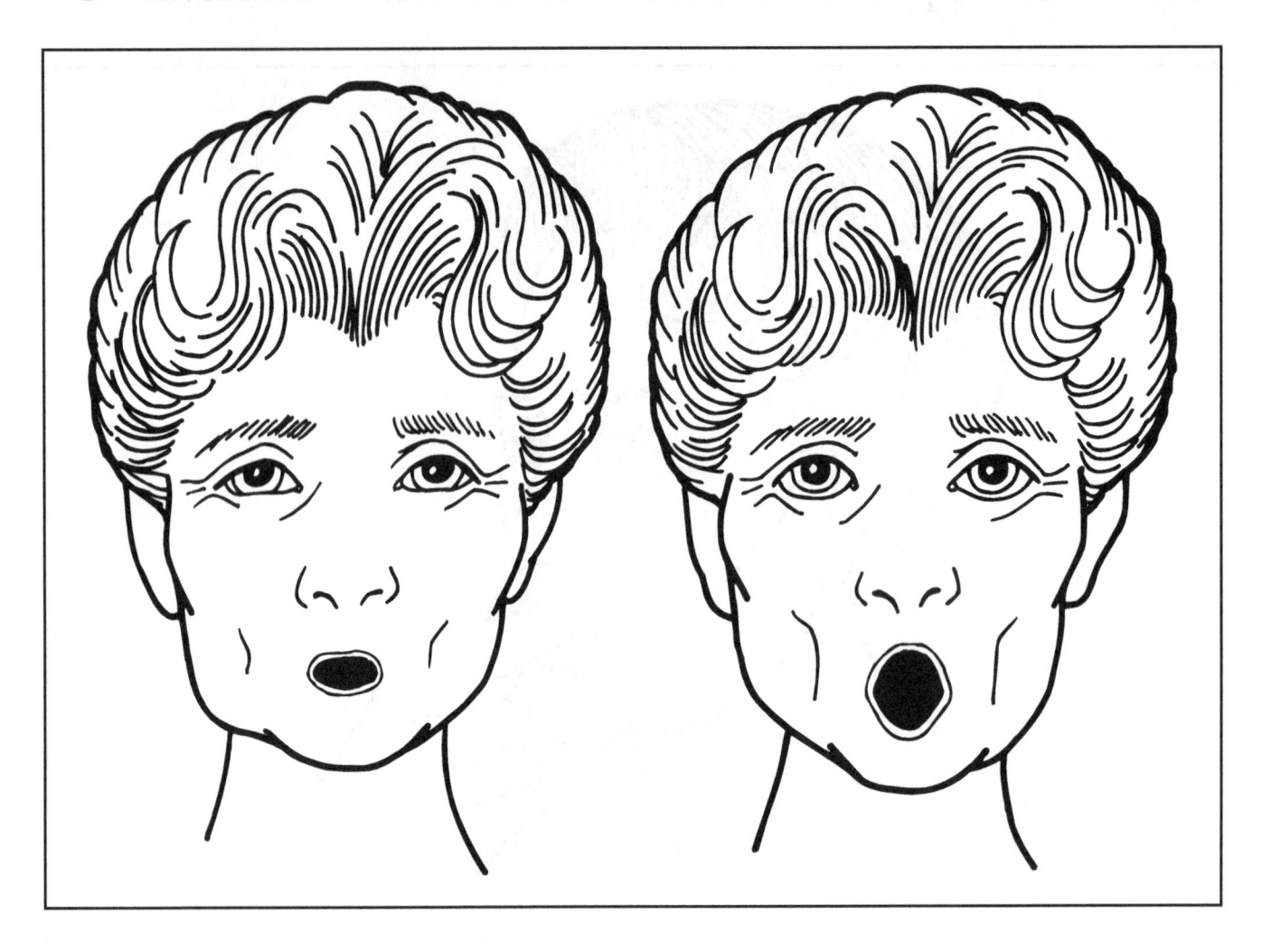

Hide lips under teeth. Purse lips in an "O." Open jaw. Pull lips inside mouth as much as possible while stretching jaw open. Relax neck muscles.

Benefits

- strengthens lips and cheeks
- improves stretch, tone, range of motion of front of lips, nose, and cheeks

Lip Curl

Chapter 10, continued

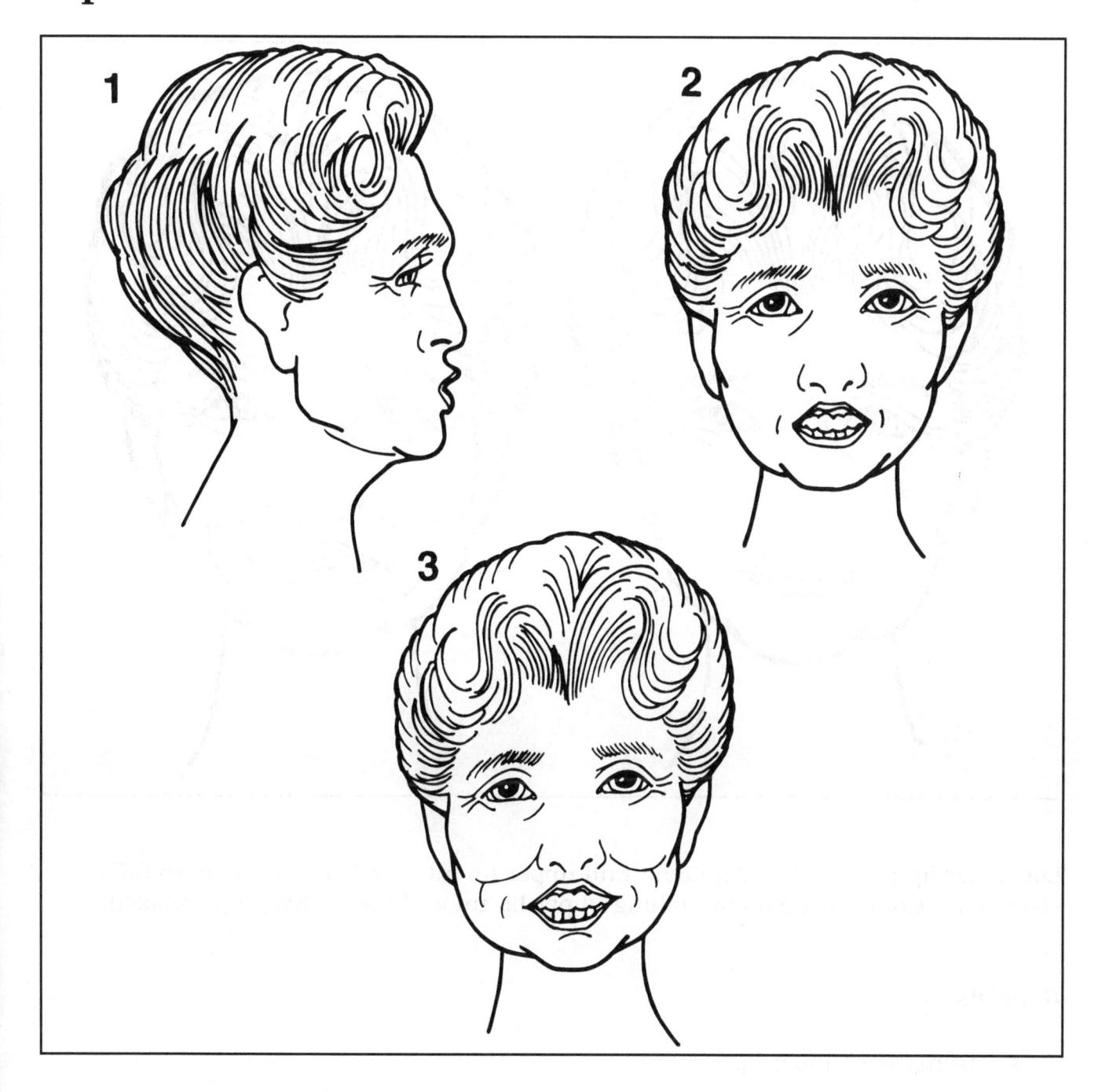

Press lips outward. Try to curl top lip upward and bottom lip downward. Maintain curl and smile.

Benefit

○ strengthens and improves range of motion of lips and cheeks

The Oral-Facial Therapy Exercise Book
2021 Edition

Upper Lip Curl

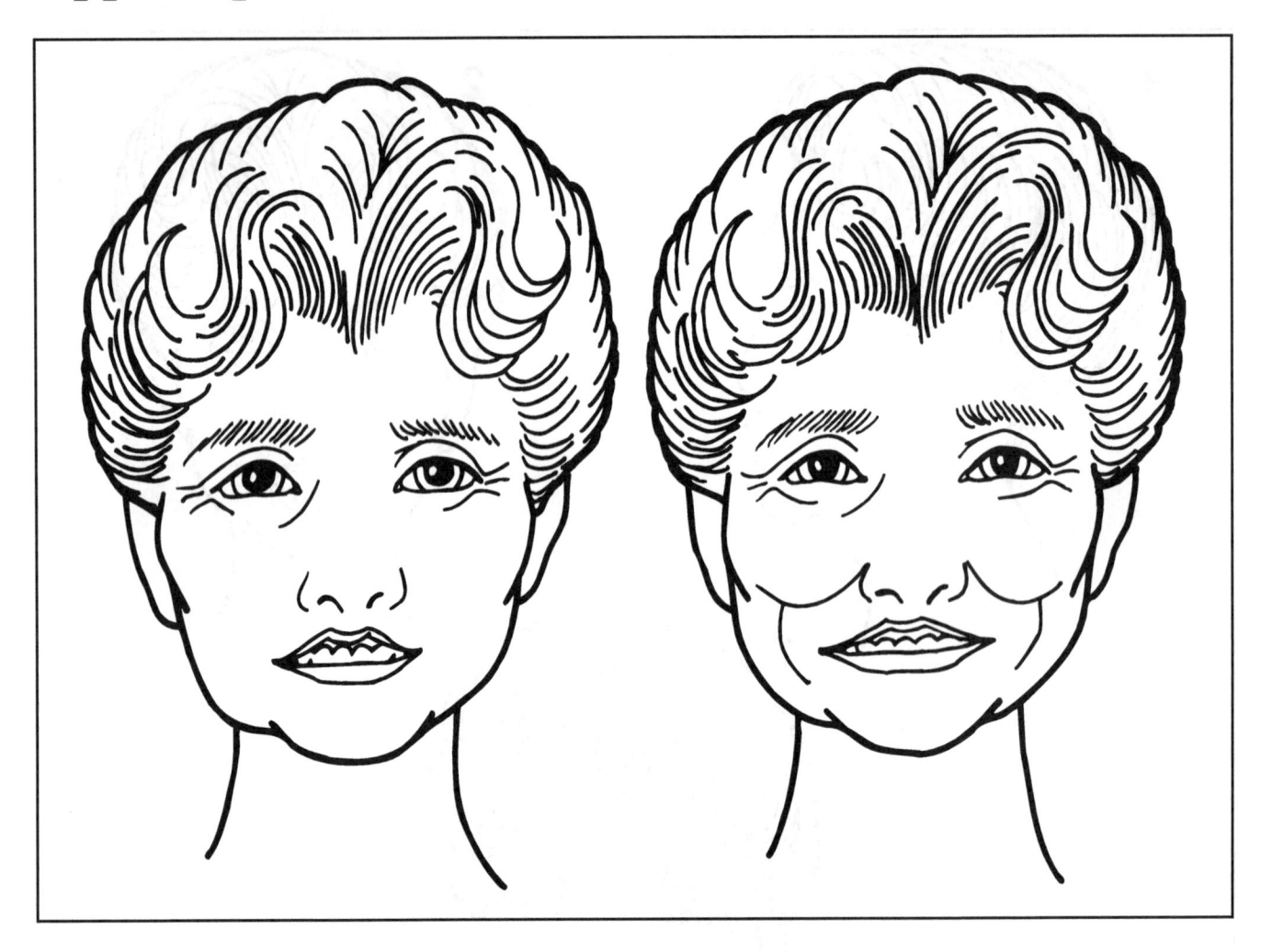

Chapter 10, continued

Lift upper lip to show the gumline. Pull upper lip into smile toward ears to full extension. Concentrate on stretching upper lip up and back. Keep jaw relaxed.

Benefits

- strengthens upper lip

- improves range of motion of upper lip

Upper Lip Exercise

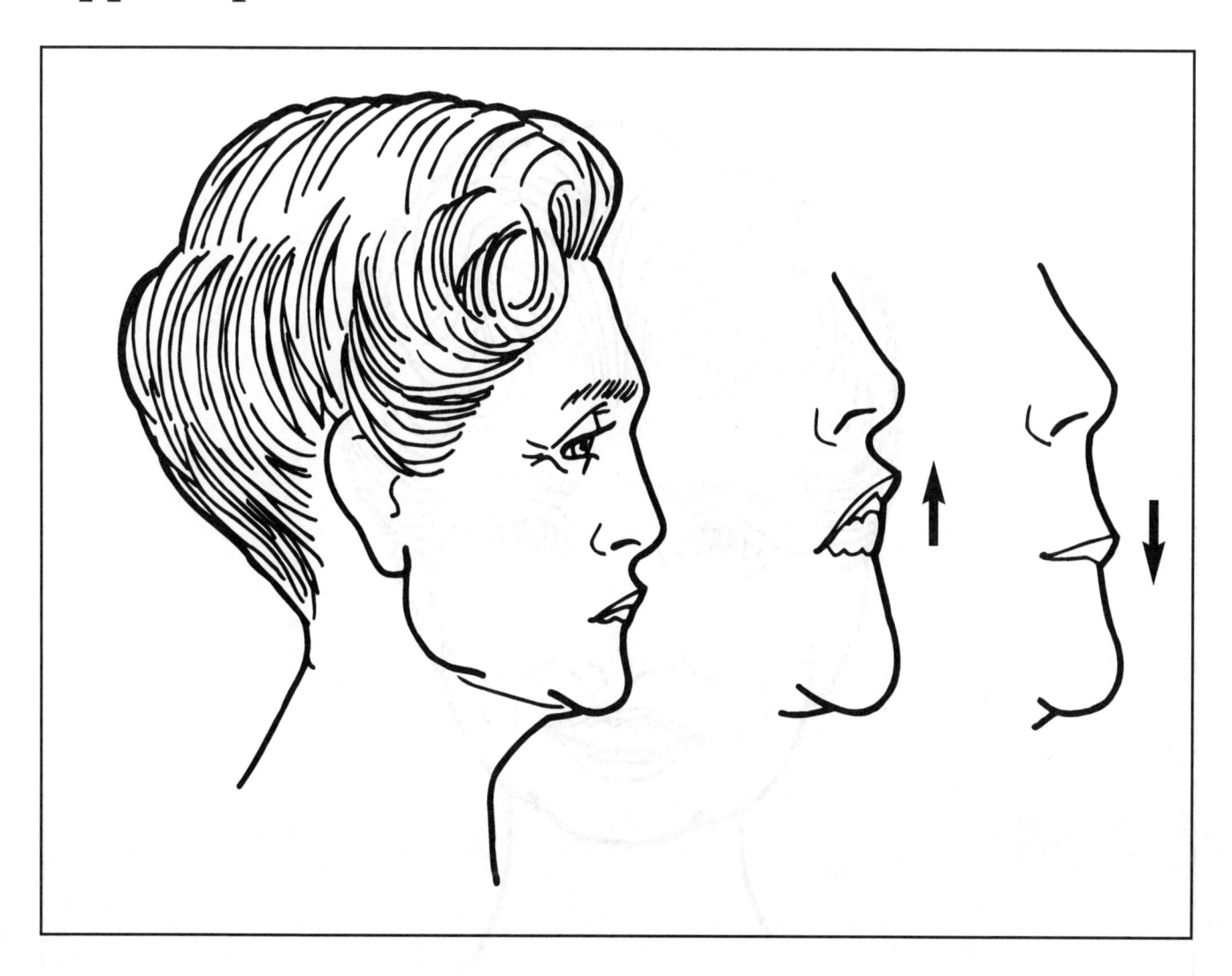

Chapter 10, continued

Bite gently on lower lip. Raise and lower upper lip. Repeat the up-and-down motion. Keep face relaxed, moving lips only. Do not squint or move your cheeks.

Benefits

- strengthens upper lip musculature
- improves range of motion and agility of upper lip

The Oral-Facial Therapy Exercise Book
2021 Edition

Smile Exercise 1

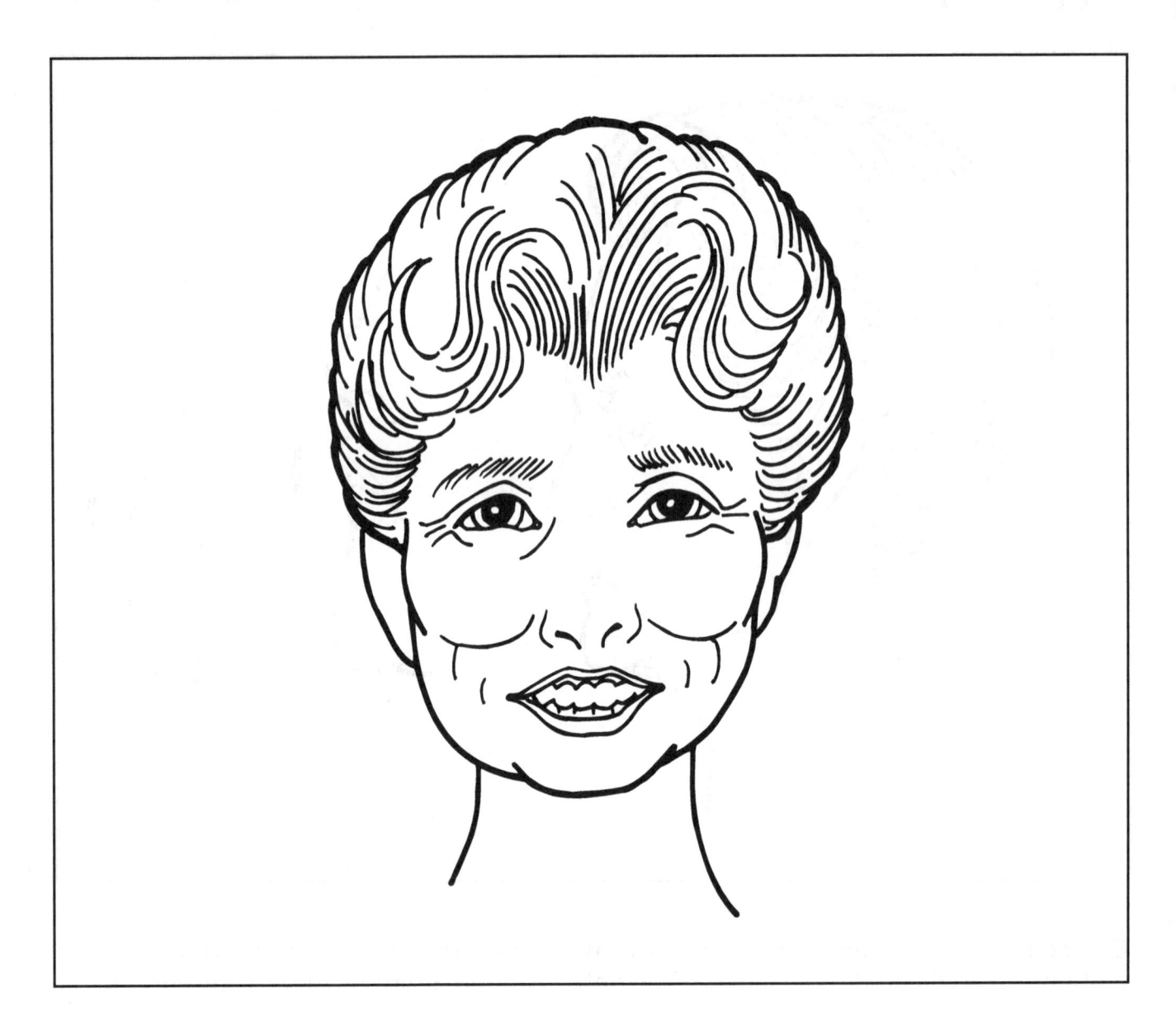

Chapter 10, continued

Smile. Show upper and lower teeth and gums in a wide grin. Clench teeth gently. Relax neck. Do not squint.

Benefits

- strengthens lips and cheeks

- stretches and improves range of motion of lips and cheeks

Smile Exercise 2

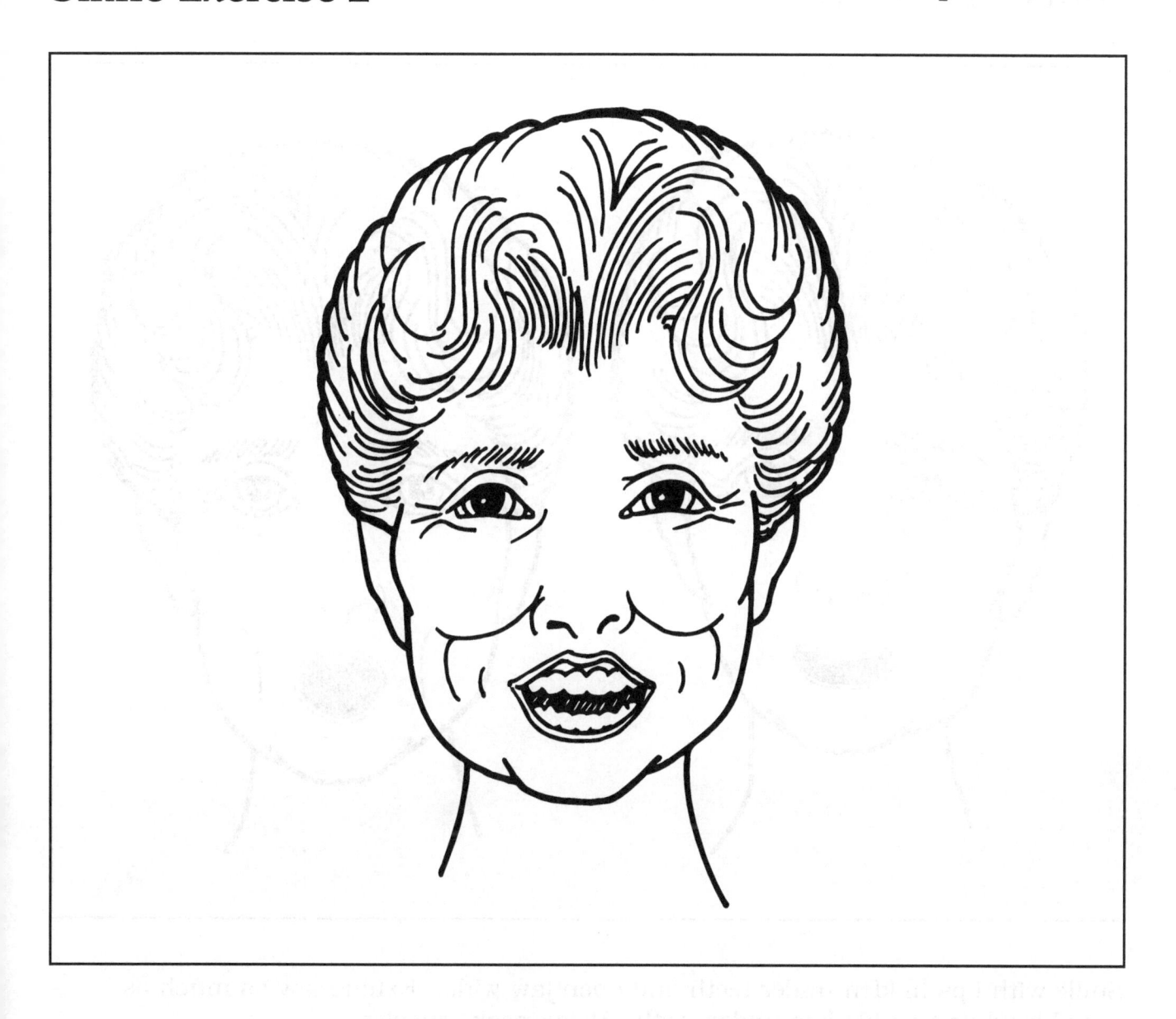

Chapter 10, *continued*

Show all upper and lower teeth in a wide grin. Open jaw. Maintain full extension of lips. Hold for 10 to 20 seconds as tolerated. Sustain for longer time as strength improves.

Benefits

- strengthens lips and cheeks

- stretches and improves range of motion of lips and cheeks

Inner Cheek Jaw Stretch

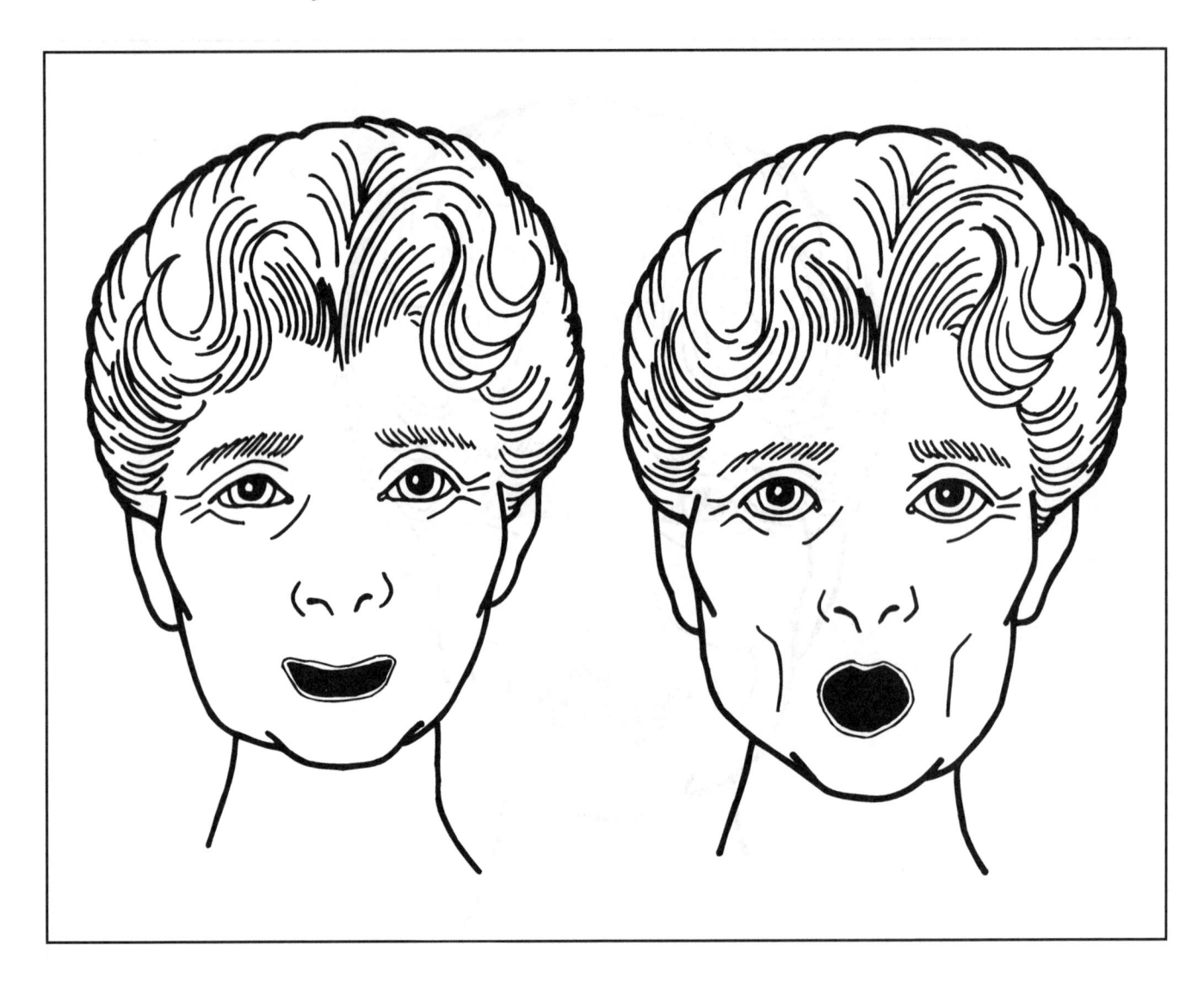

Chapter 10, continued

Smile with lips hidden under teeth and open jaw wide. Extend jaw as much as possible while keeping lips under teeth. Relax neck muscles.

Benefit

○ stretches and tones inner cheeks, jaw, and lips

Lip and Cheek Stretch

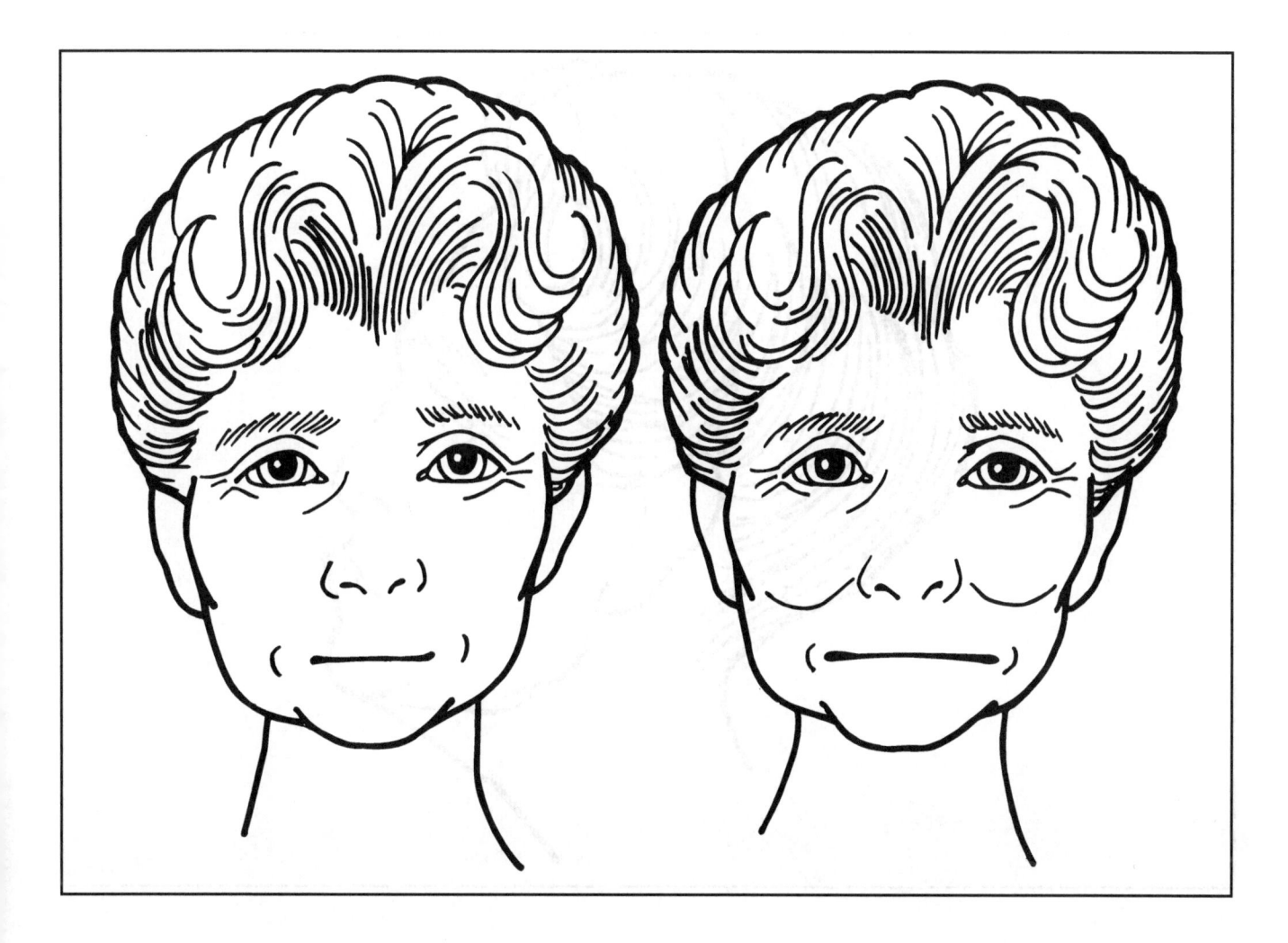

Chapter 10, continued

Hide lips under teeth. Keep mouth closed and pull lips in a straight line. Stretch lip corners toward jaw. Stretch as wide as possible, maintaining a closed mouth. Then smile wide with a closed mouth. Relax neck muscles.

Benefits

- strengthens lips and cheeks

- improves range of motion of lips and cheeks

The Oral-Facial Therapy Exercise Book
2021 Edition

Lower Lip Extension

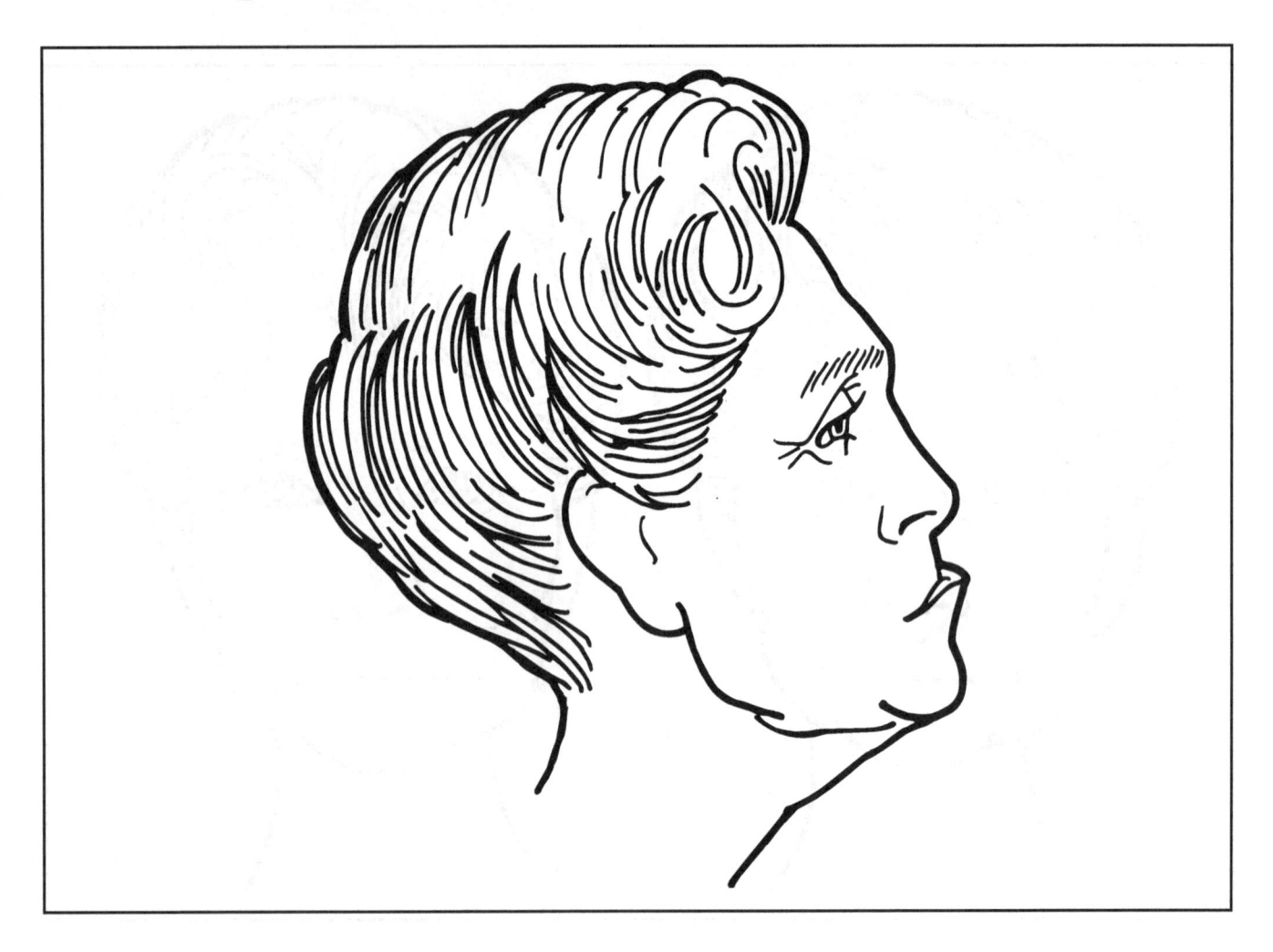

Chapter 10, continued

Lift lower lip up. Hold to full extension. To also work neck, raise head upward and hold.

Benefits

- strengthens lower lip

- stretches and tones neck

- improves range of motion of lip and chin musculature

Lip Press

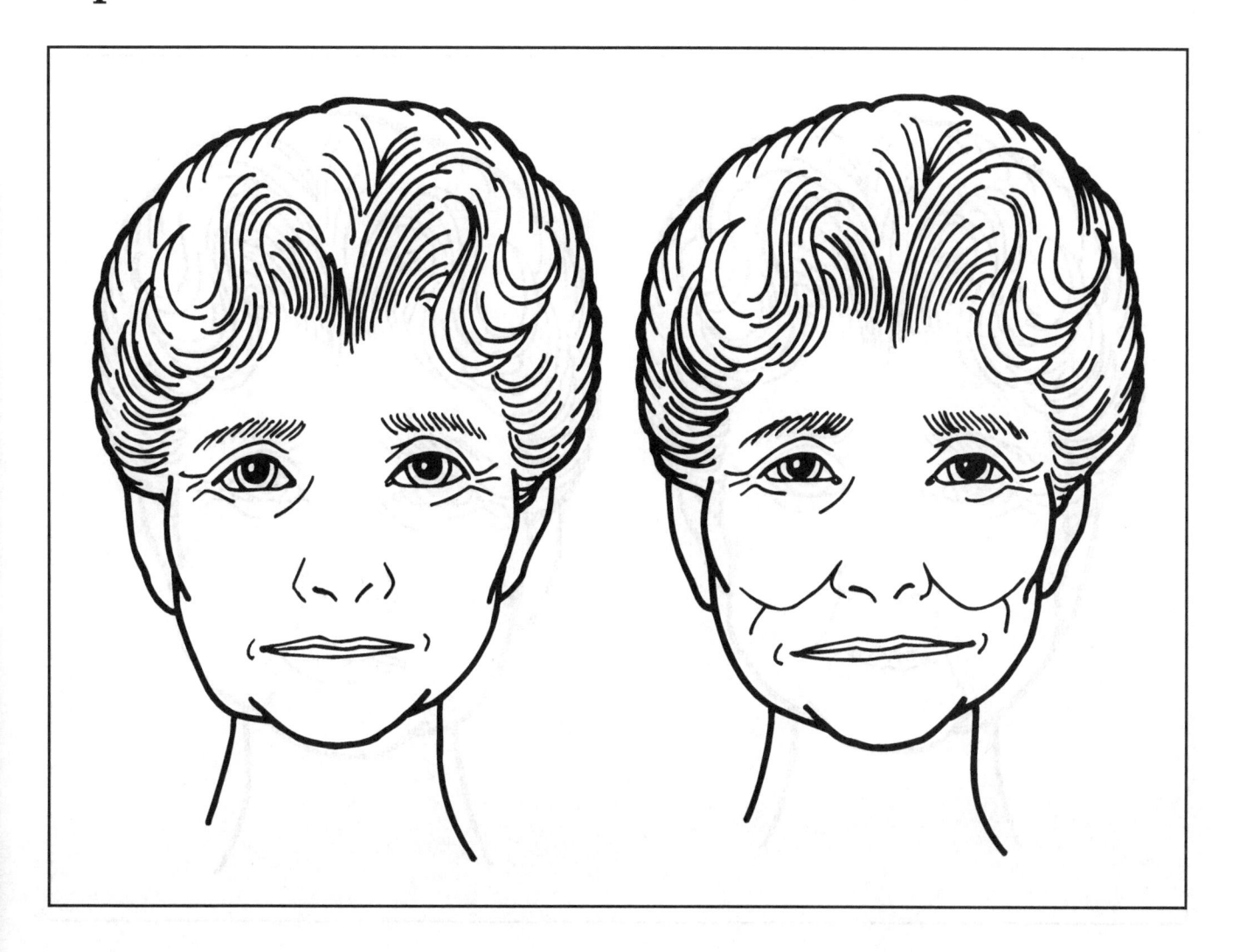

Chapter 10, *continued*

Press lips together firmly and evenly. Keep lips pressed together and begin to smile. Broaden smile to full extension. Use equal pressure with both lips.

Benefits

- strengthens lips and cheek musculature
- improves range of motion of lips and cheeks

Cheek Puff/Lip Purse

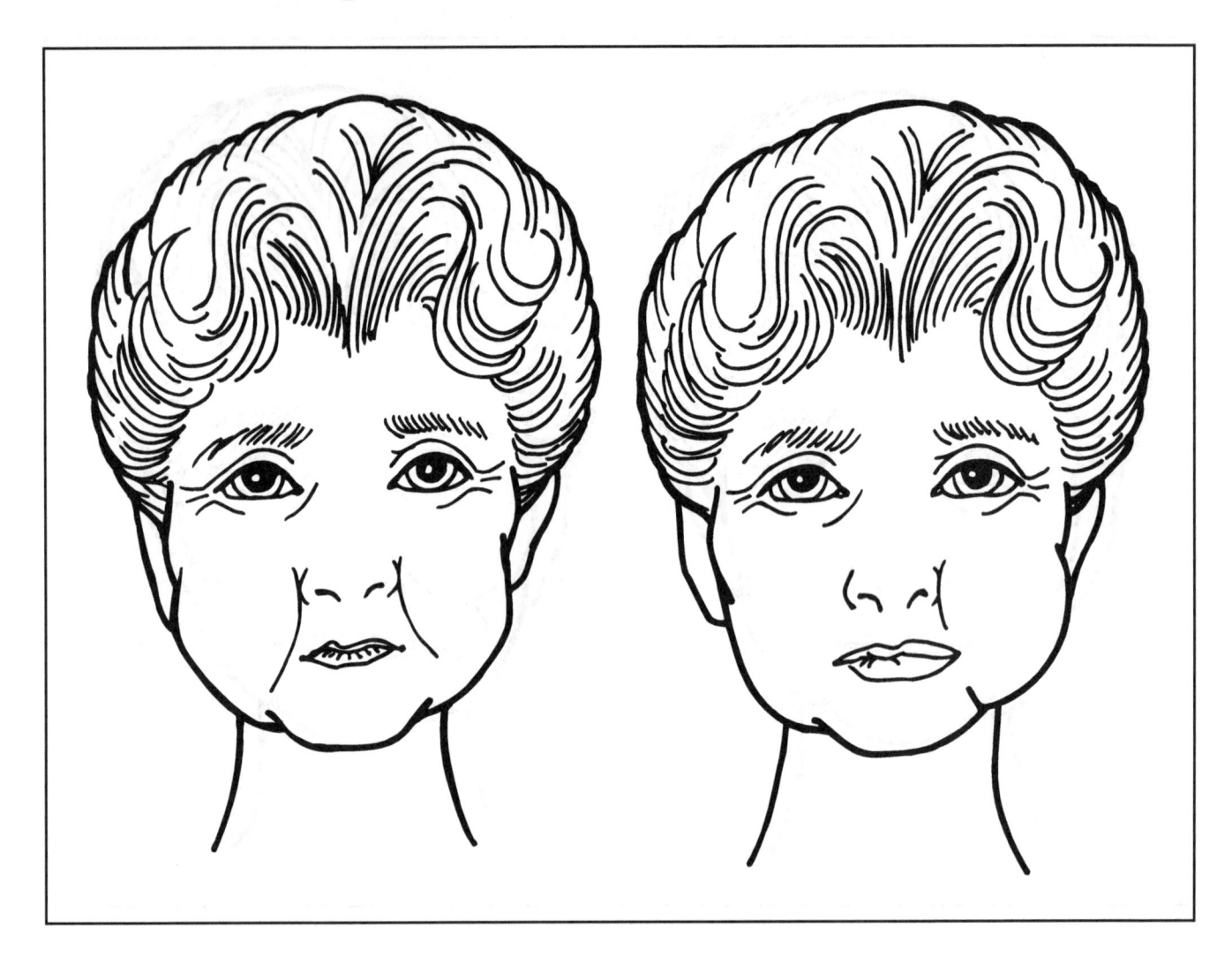

Chapter 10, continued

Puff out cheeks with securely pursed lips. Hold air in puffed-out cheeks. Do not let air out of nose or lips. For added difficulty, hold air in left cheek only. Then switch to right cheek only.

Benefits

- strengthens lip pursing

- stretches and tones cheeks

Lip and Cheek Toner

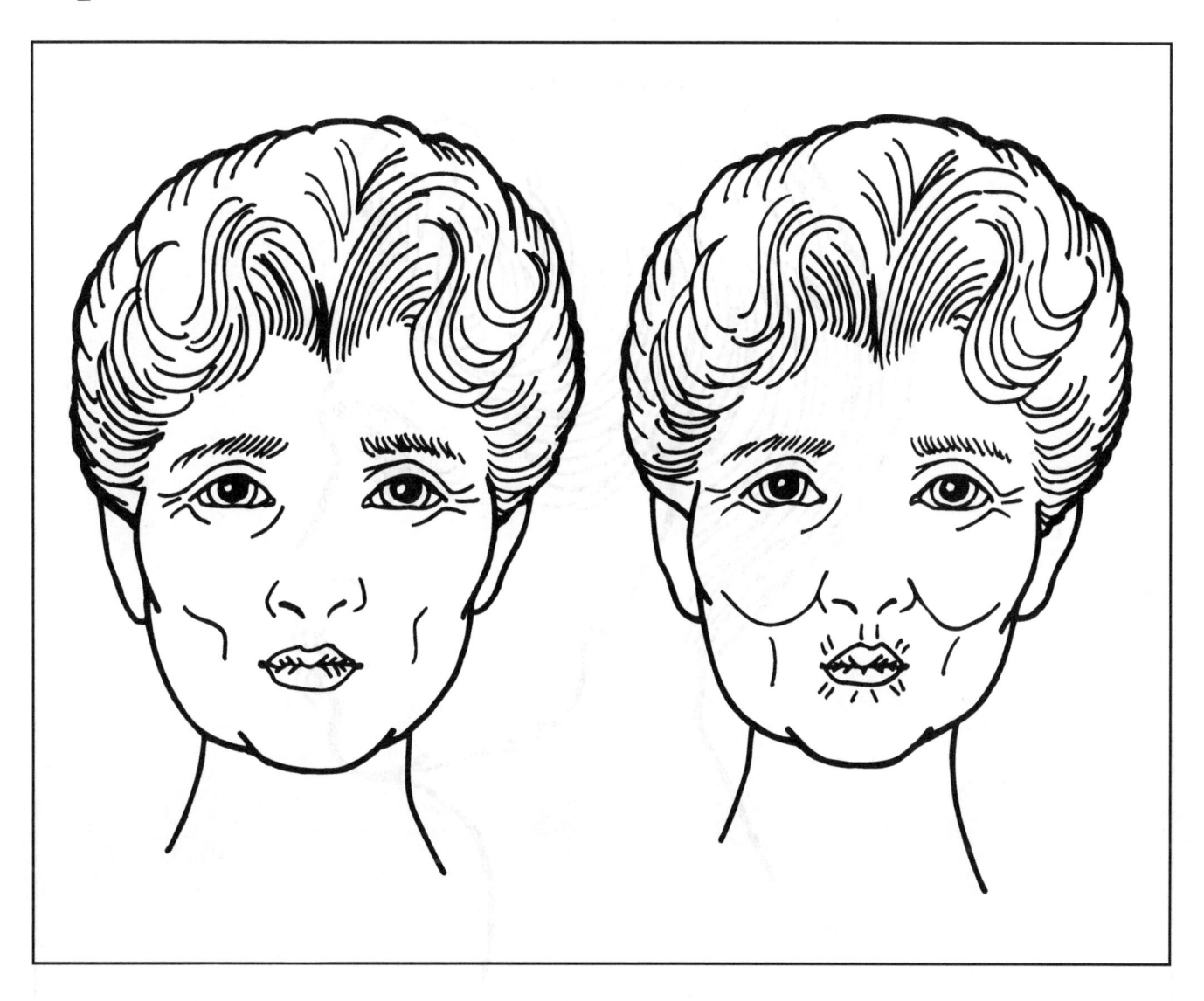

Chapter 10, *continued*

Close lips. Pretend to suck on a straw, but keep lips closed. Suck in inner cheeks. Maintain suction in mouth. Relax neck. For added difficulty, raise cheeks in a smiling manner.

Benefit

○ strengthens and tones lips and cheeks

Lip Vibration

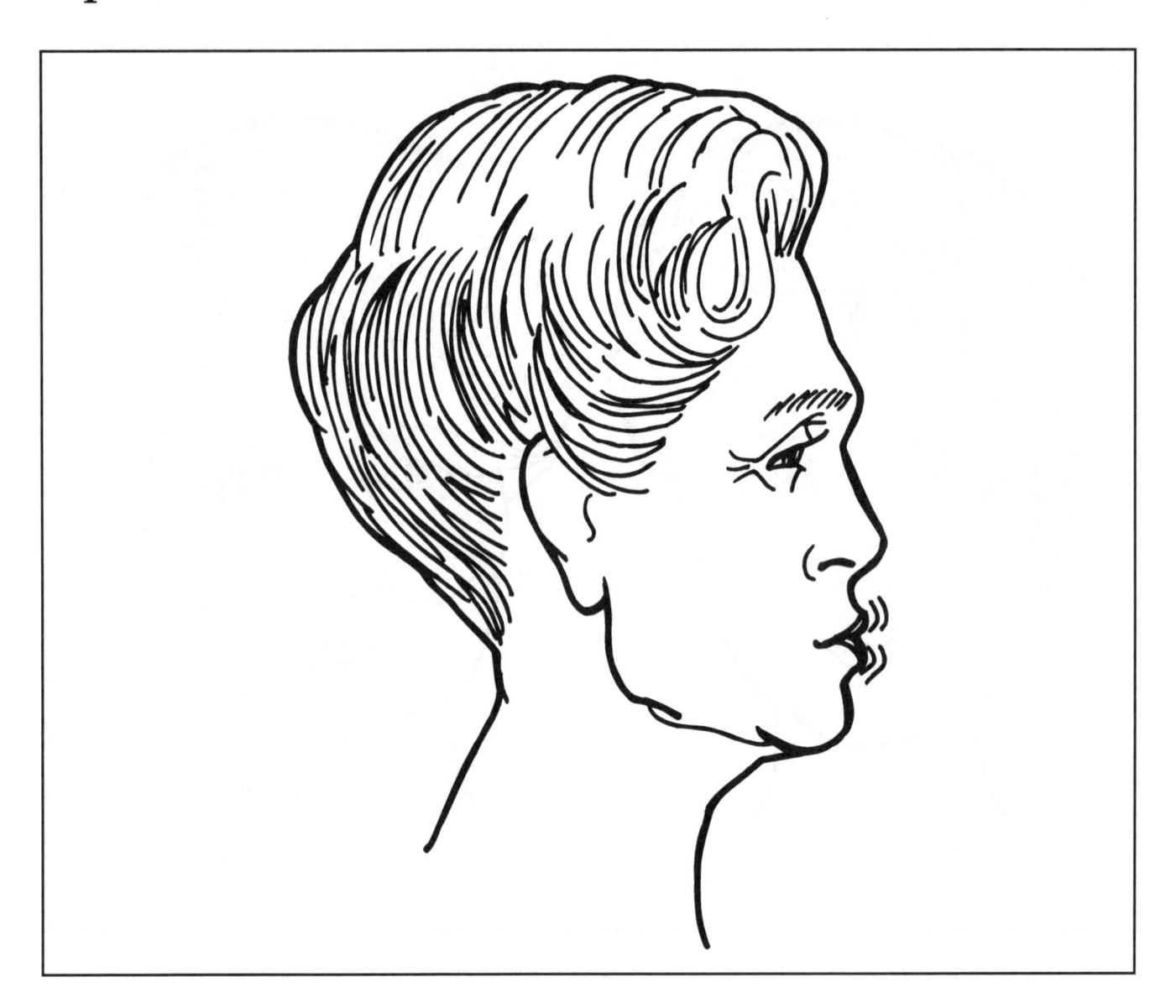

Chapter 10, continued

Exhale air through slightly pursed lips, allowing vibration to occur.

Benefit

- strengthens inner lips

Full-Face Scrunch

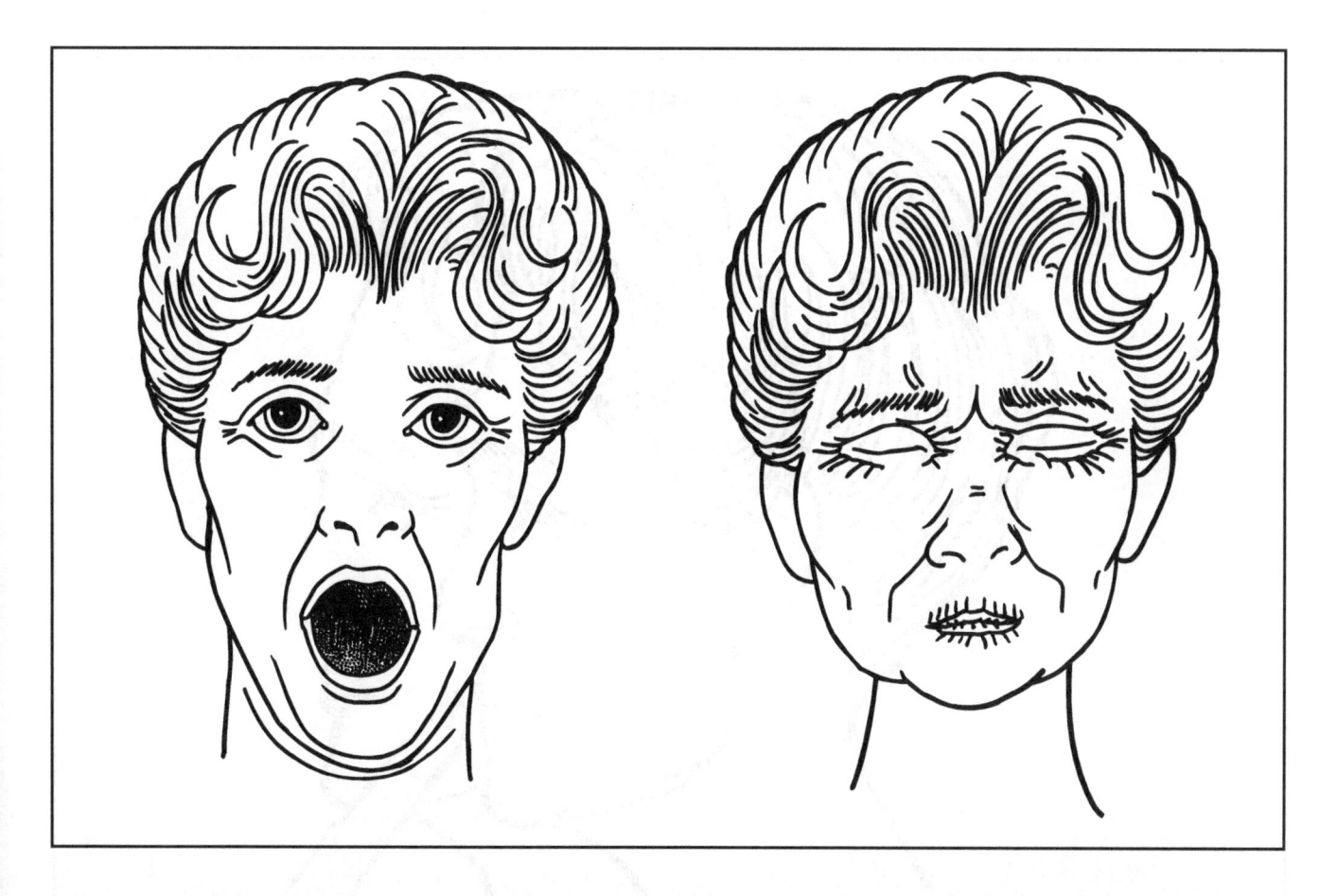

Chapter 10, continued

Have the client stretch and contract her facial musculature several times using different examples and visuals.

1. Have the client make a wide-open expression of surprise. Then have the client scrunch up her face hard.

2. Tell the client to pretend she is trying to make a baby smile and to over-exaggerate a wide-open expression of amazement. Then ask her to make the baby laugh by scrunching up her face as much as possible.

3. Say, "Make your face 3 times smaller than it is." Then say, "Make your face 5 times bigger than it is."

Keep going back and forth to stretch and contract the facial musculature. Try to have the client hold each expression for a few seconds before releasing to the other expression.

> Note: This is an excellent exercise for the ocular area (around the eyes), the forehead, the nose, the cheeks, the jaw, and the lips. It will also help to stretch and strengthen the neck. It's fun and a great way to energize the individual.

Upper Lip Movement

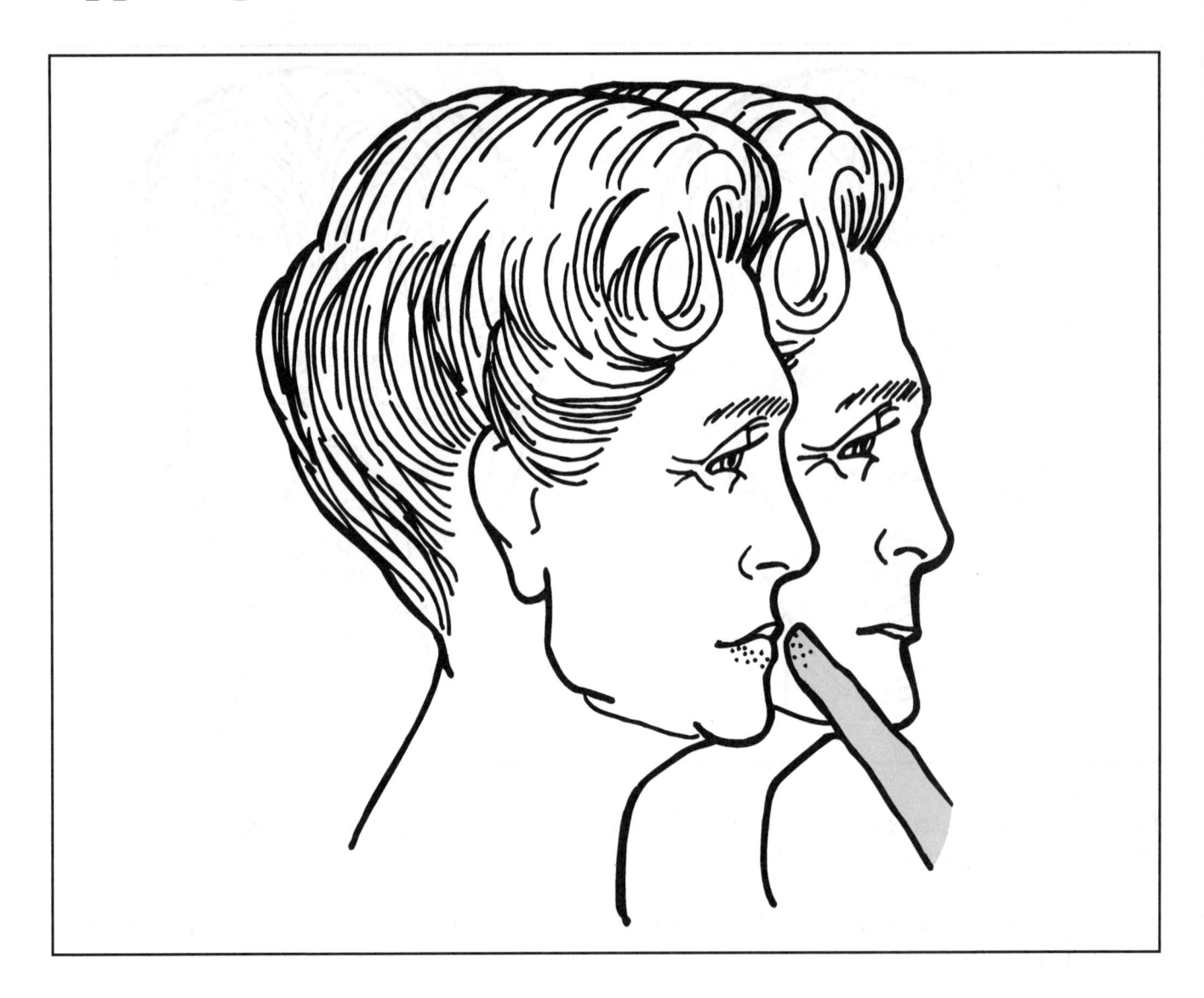

Chapter 10, continued

Lightly tap with the tip of the finger the outer edge of lower lip. Then demonstrate and have the client stretch and cover the area you tapped with the upper lip. Encourage upper lip stretching down to cover.

Benefits

- ○ reduces drooling

- ○ strengthens lips

The Oral-Facial Therapy Exercise Book
2021 Edition

Lip Hold

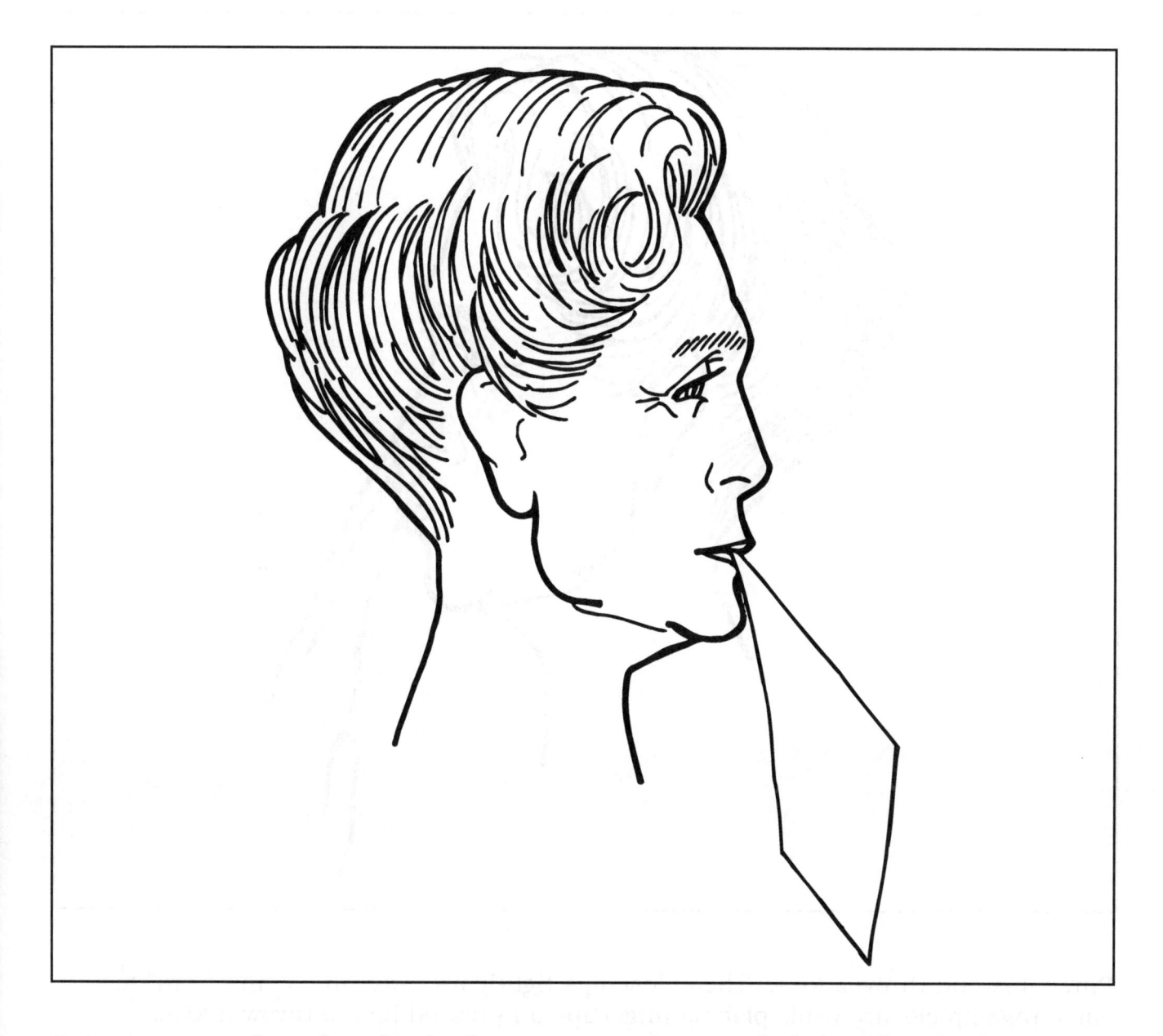

Chapter 10, *continued*

Put a corner edge of a sheet of paper, a napkin, a cloth handkerchief, or a washcloth between lips. Press firmly with lips only. Hold in place 20 seconds.

Benefits

- reduces drooling

- strengthens lips and inner cheeks

The Oral-Facial Therapy Exercise Book
2021 Edition

Kissing Exercise

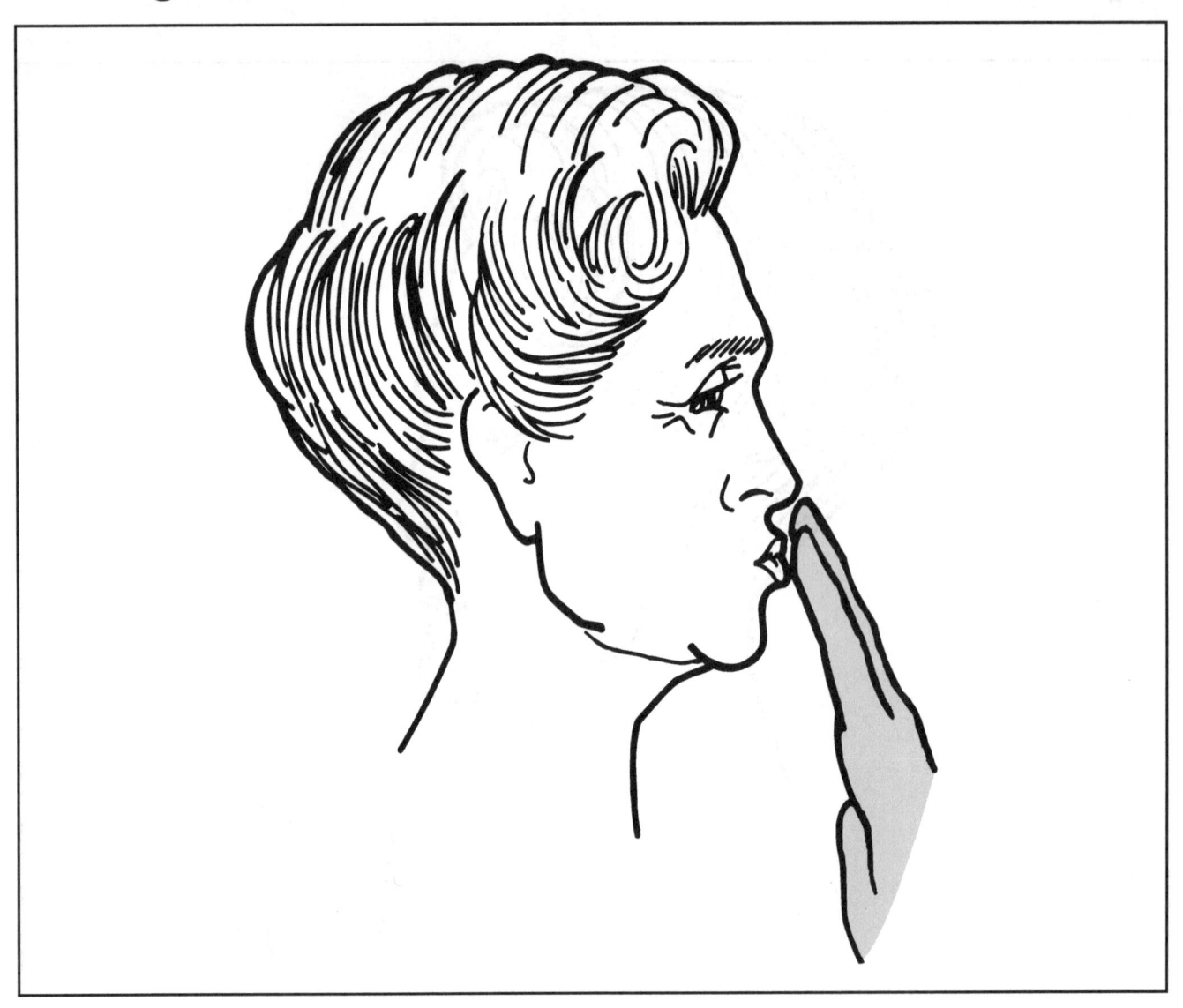

Chapter 10, continued

Purse lips and throw a kiss. Then close lips tightly and say "m . . . m . . . m" to encourage lip closure while placing fingertips on pressed lips to throw a kiss.

For additional practice, produce the sounds /m/, /p/, and /b/ to encourage lip closure. Start with "me . . . me . . . me." Concentrate on tightening the lips. Then say "pea . . . pea . . . pea . . ." and "bee . . . bee . . . bee . . .".

Benefits

- improves lip pursing
- assists in pre-speech formation of /m, p, b/

Upper Lip Squeeze

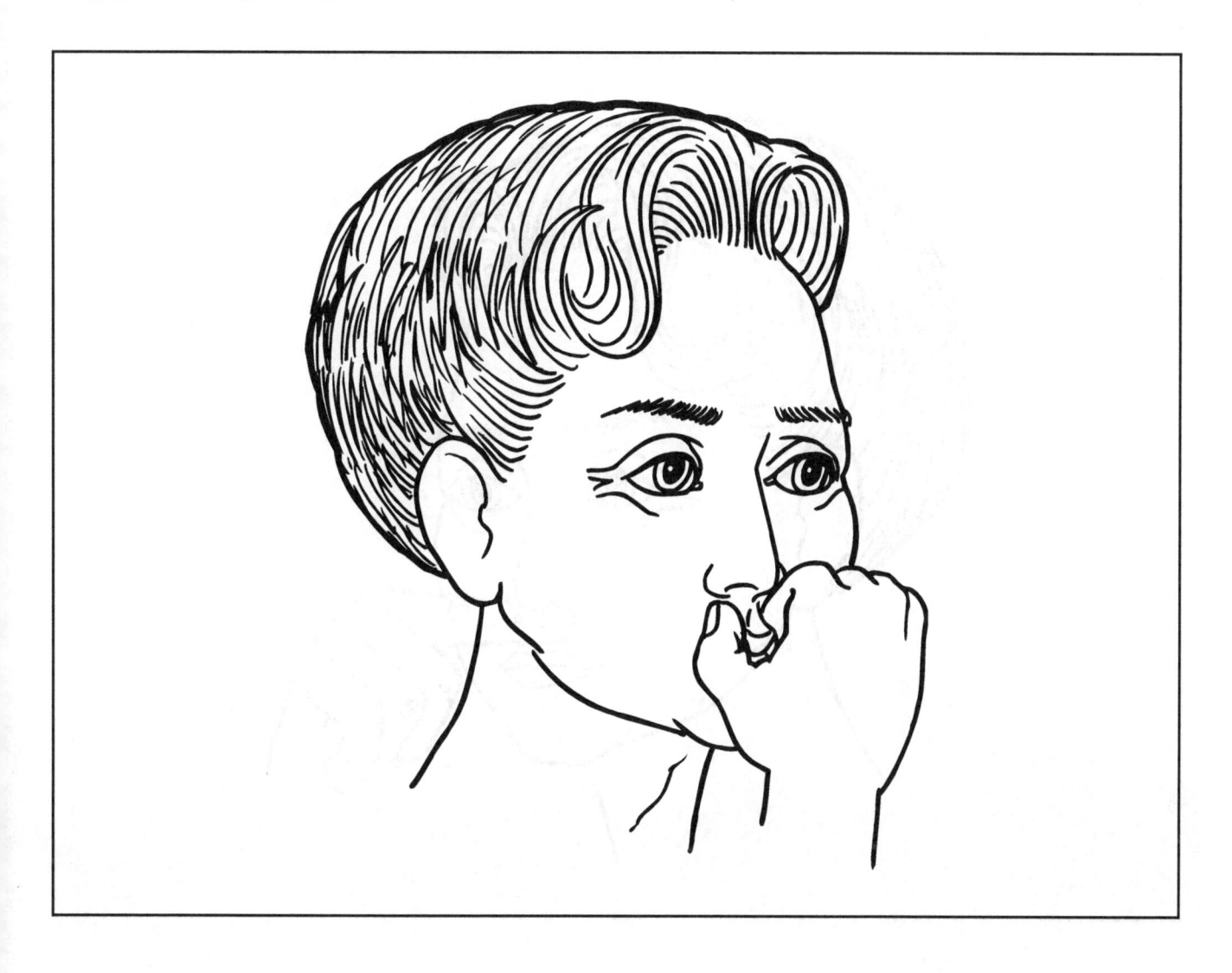

Chapter 10, continued

Gently grasp upper lip under the bridge of the nose with the index finger and thumb. Apply pressure for 30 seconds. Then lightly squeeze and gently massage musculature under the skin.

Benefits

- stretches and elongates upper lip to form a seal for /p, b, m/
- stimulates downward motion of lip to improve swallowing and reduce drooling

Upper Lip Stretch — Middle

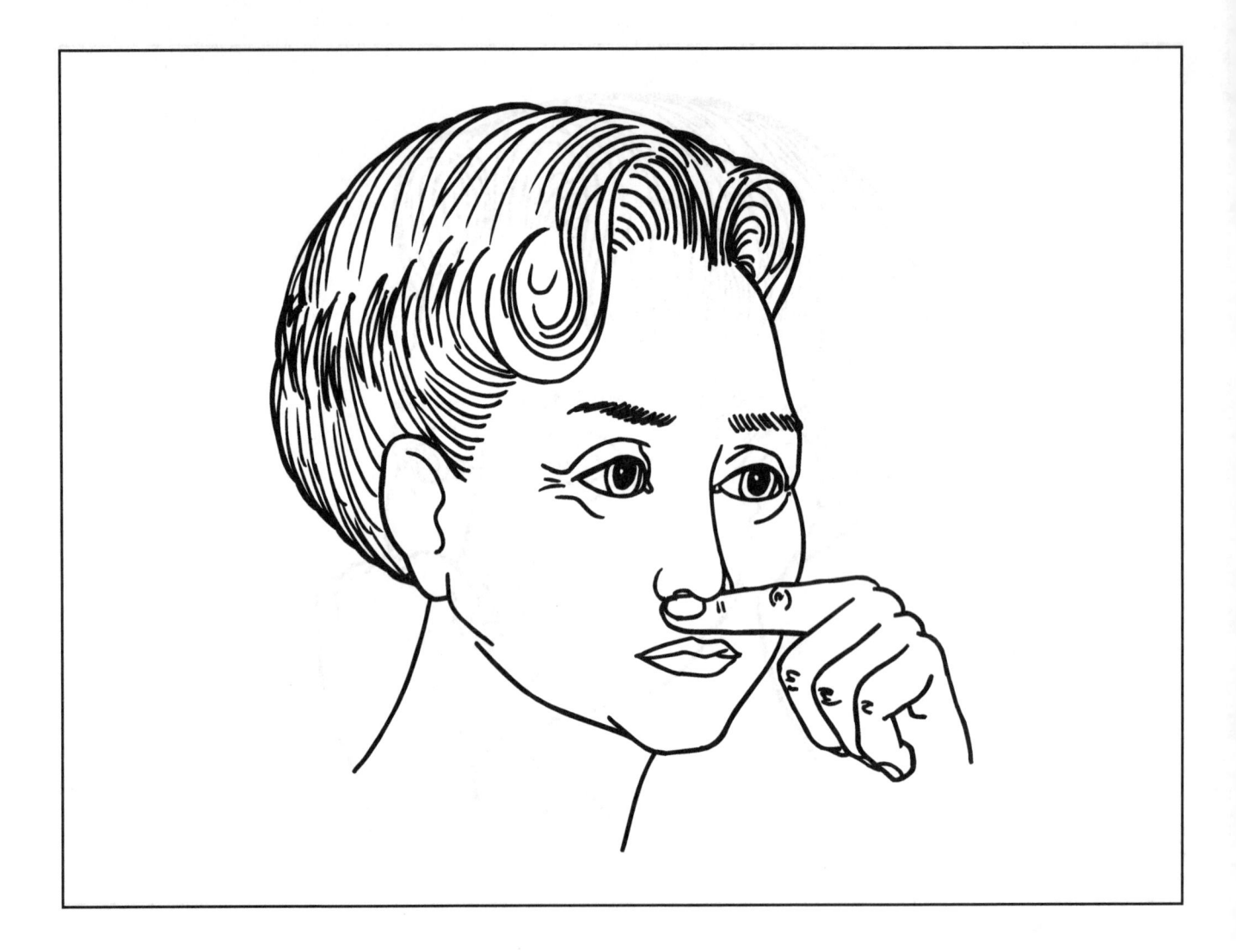

Chapter 10, continued

Place index finger horizontally over upper lip. Tuck side of finger up against the base of nose. Apply gentle pressure and roll the finger down toward the lip. Repeat 5 times.

Benefits

- relieves tension in upper lip and nasal area

- assists in stretching and toning the upper lip to form a seal for improved swallowing and speech production

Assisted Raspberry

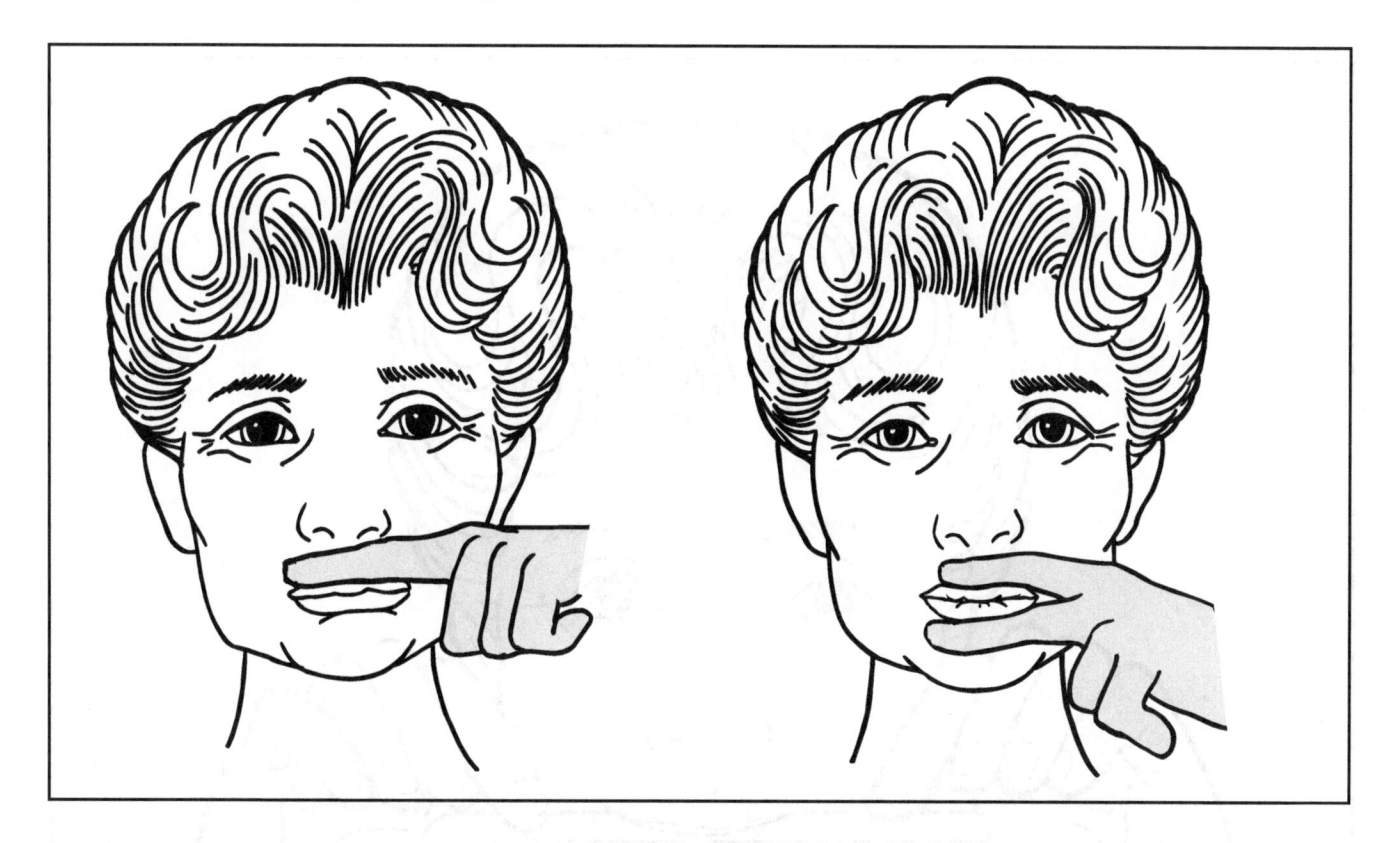

Chapter 10, continued

To determine if the client's lips are too weak to self-initiate and/or maintain a lip seal, have the client try to make a raspberry or buzzing noise with her lips. If she is not able to do it, put your index finger horizontally across her upper lip. Push it downward and ask the individual to take a deep breath and blow. If vibration is produced, try again but offer slightly less assistance. Continue offering less and less assistance until the lips and cheeks are strengthened for an improved lip seal.

If pushing down the upper lip does not create a seal sufficient for a bit of vibration, place your middle finger horizontally under the client's lower lip. Push her lips together and again ask her to take a deep breath and blow hard. If vibration is produced, repeat. Offer less and less assistance over time to strengthen the lips and cheeks.

Benefits

- builds tone and strength for lip seal for improved swallowing and speech production

- reduces drooling

Horizontal Lip Strengthener

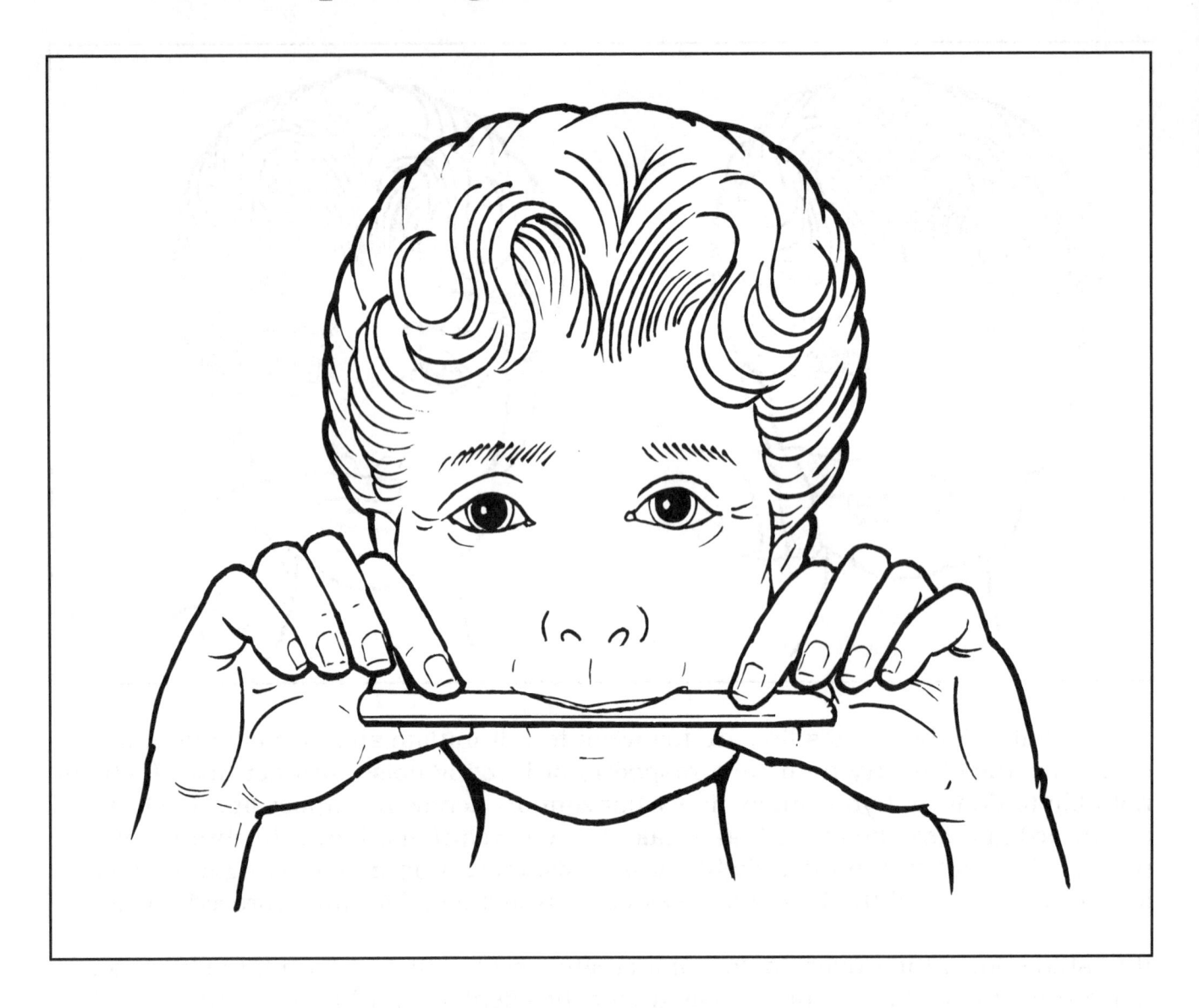

Chapter 10, continued

Place a tongue depressor or Popsicle stick horizontally between the lips only. Pull out gently on the stick with equal effort on each end to offer resistance to the lips. Start out offering very little resistance, then build up as the lips grow stronger.

Benefits

- improves lip seal and lip rounding
- strengthens inner cheeks and neck musculature

Rounded Lip Strengthener

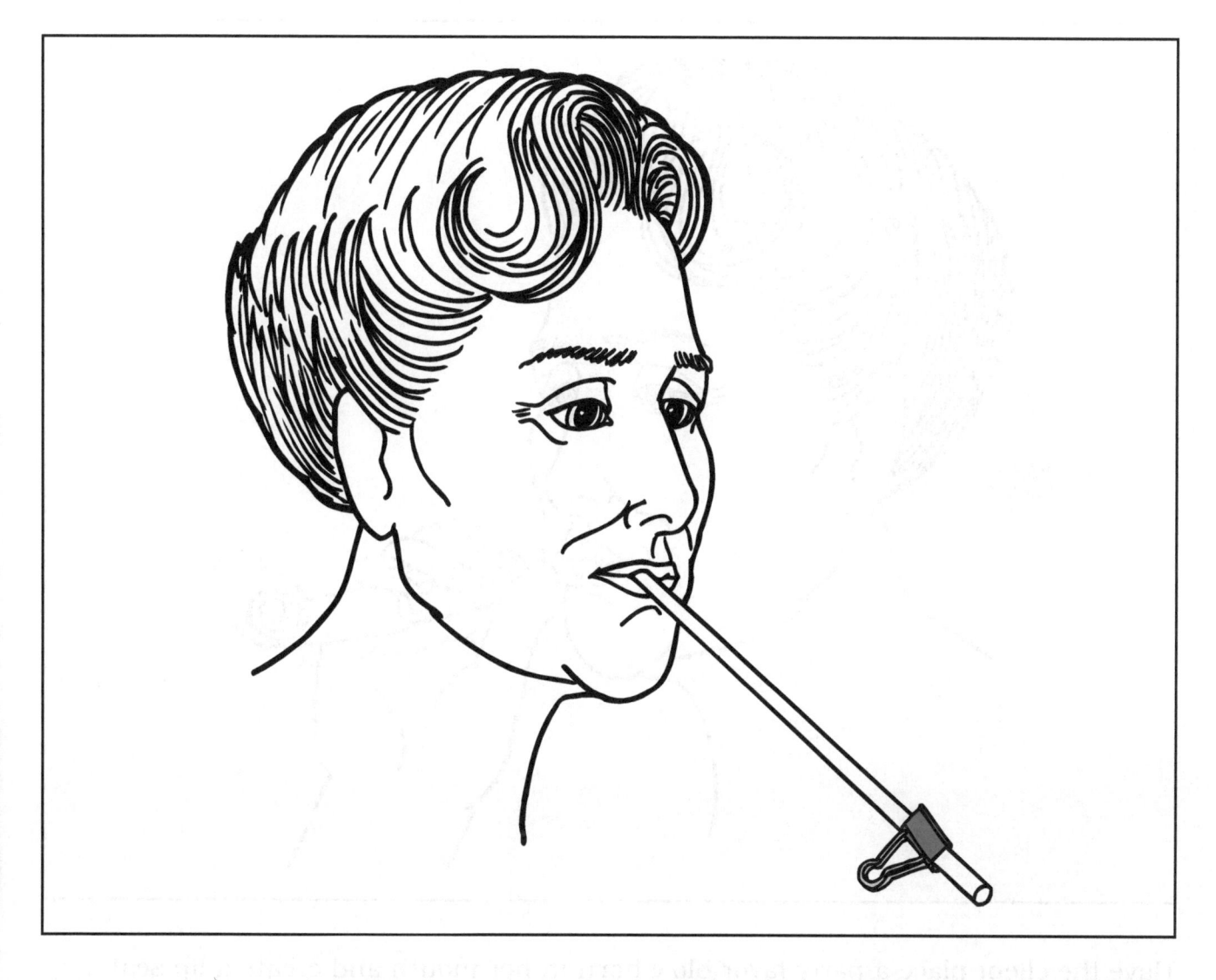

Chapter 10, continued

Place the end of a straw in the client's mouth, having her hold it with the lips only. Offer less and less support until the individual is able to support the weight of the straw on her own.

To add further weight, attach a paper clip to the extended end of the straw. As the client grasps the straw, ask her to push it up with her lips so that it sticks out of her mouth horizontally. Remind the client to keep her head still, her teeth closed and to only use her lips.

Benefit

- strengthens cheeks, chin, and lips

Party Favor

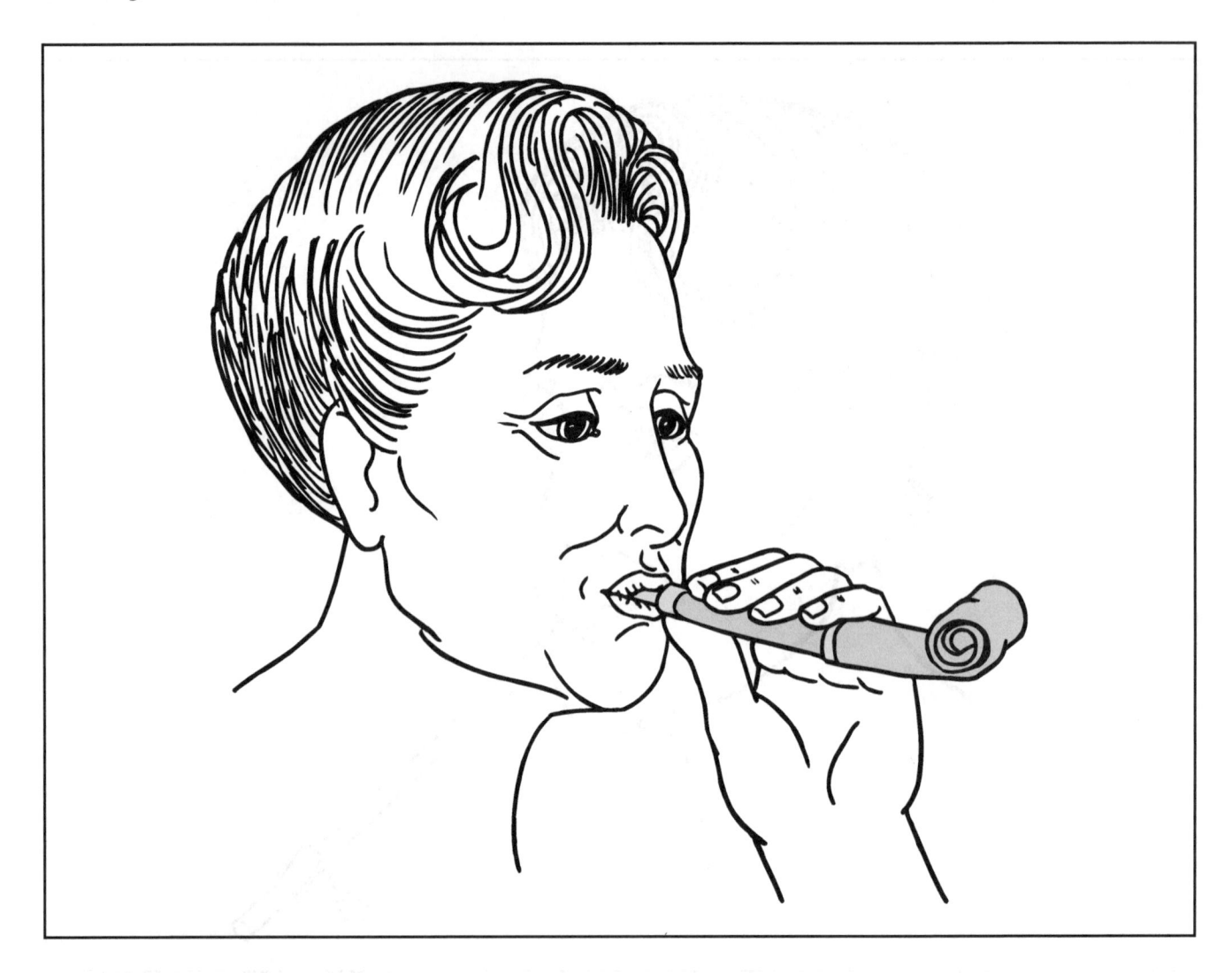

Chapter 10, continued

Have the client place a party favor blow horn in her mouth and create a lip seal around it. (You might need to use your index finger and thumb around the individual's lips to help create a seal.) Ask the client to blow hard. Repeat the action three times.

Note: If the client is having difficulty creating a lip seal, practice additional lip exercises provided.

Benefit

○ strengthens and tones outer and inner lip seal and inner cheek muscles

The Oral-Facial Therapy Exercise Book
2021 Edition

Lip Frenulum Stretch

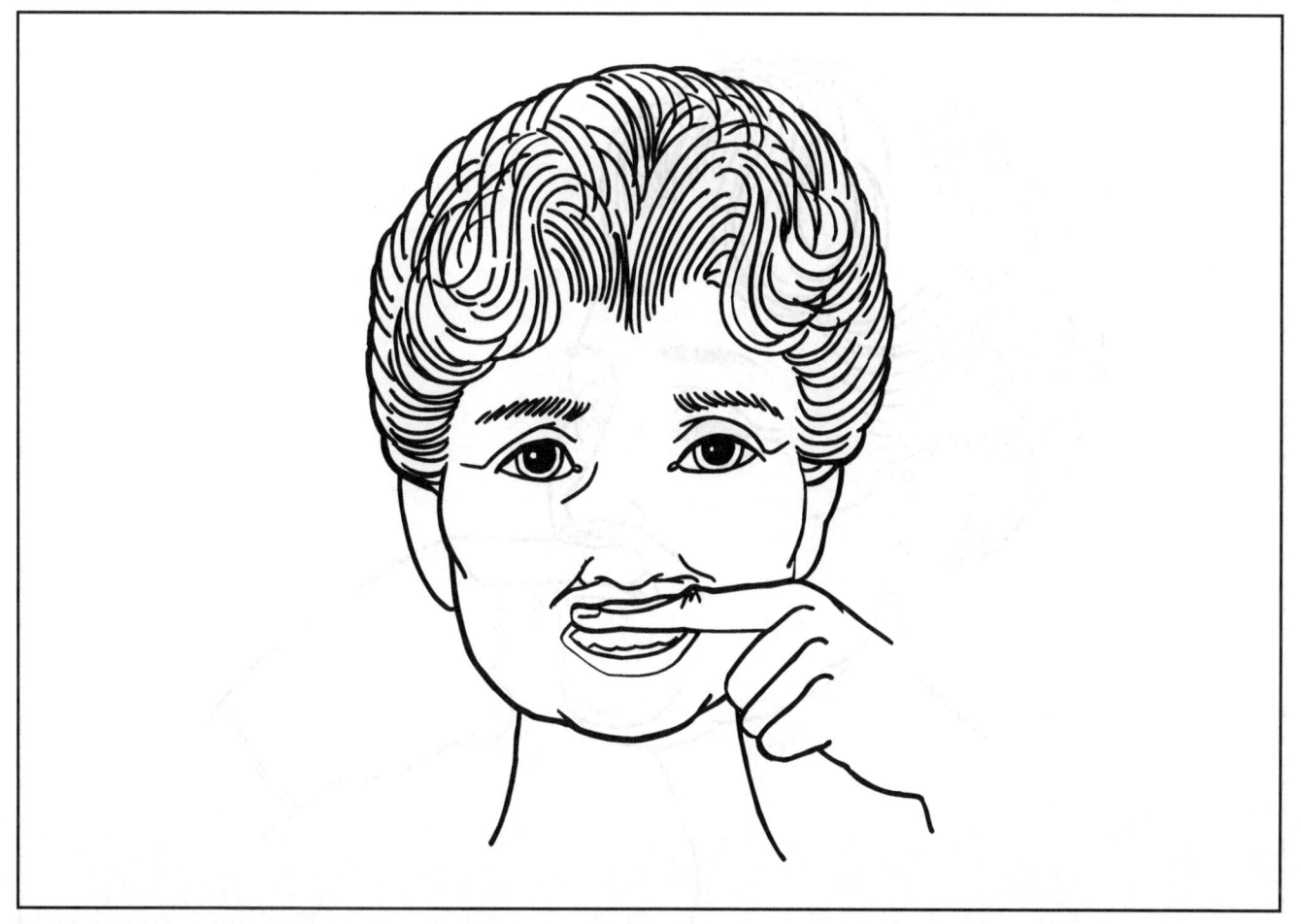

Chapter 10, continued

A restrictive frenulum can interfere with lip approximation for articulation. Daily stretching of the frenulum will free it from the gum and upper lip allowing greater range of motion.

Place flat side of index finger against the inner upper lip and push up against the gums. Apply moderate pressure as tolerated and hold for 30 seconds. Repeat three times.

Use the same technique for lower lip if the frenulum is restricting lower lip range of motion.

Benefits

- increases lip range of motion
- improves lip closure

The Oral-Facial Therapy Exercise Book
2021 Edition

Lower Lip Strengthener

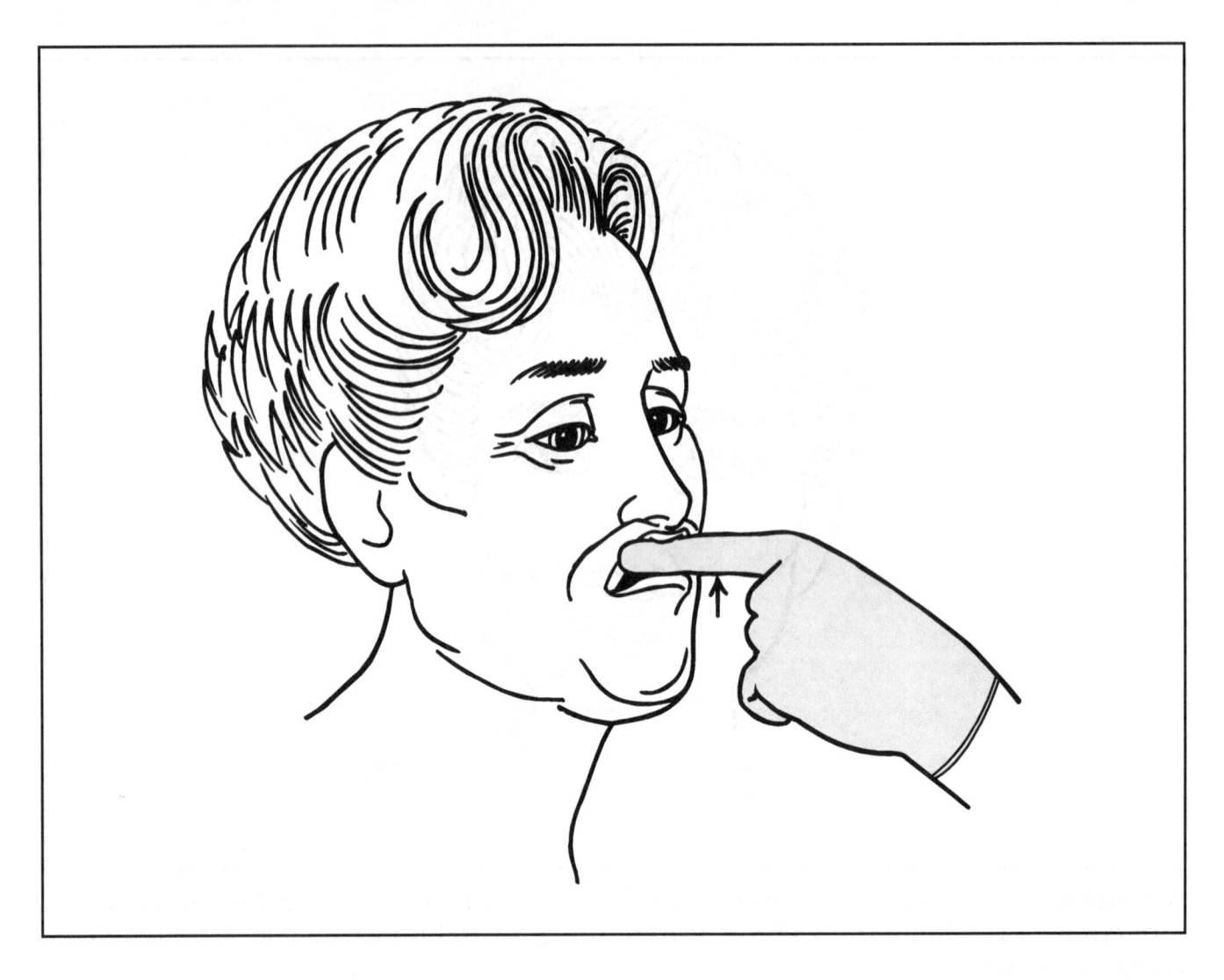

Chapter 10, continued

Hold upper lip up with index finger. Attempt to bring lower lip up to upper lip. Keep cheeks relaxed so the lower lip has a chance to strengthen.

Benefit

○ stretches and strengthens lower lip to help it form closure with the upper lip

More Lip and Cheek Exercises

Chapter 10, continued

Chew Exercise

To build inner cheek tone in mild to moderate weakness, have the client smile, bite down on teeth, and maintain clench throughout the exercise. Squeeze cheeks hard while having the client say "chew" until lips end in a pursed position. Start with a tensed smile, and end with pursed lips as the word "chew" is uttered.

Whistling

Whistling will also strengthen inner cheek musculature and inner lip pursing. Have the client whistle a favorite song or silently count to 50, making a short whistle on each number. For the client who is unable to make a whistling sound, the exercise is still beneficial in promoting cheek and lip musculature.

> Note: Encourage the individual to breathe, sigh, and express whatever comes to mind. Exercises are a stimulator for speech production, sensory awareness, and a release of feelings and emotions. Listen and respond attentively with empathy. Ask, "How are you doing?" Sometimes blocked musculature will release a wave of tingles or warmth to arms, fingers, face, feet, or belly.

Chapter 11: Tongue Exercises

Downward Tongue Stretch

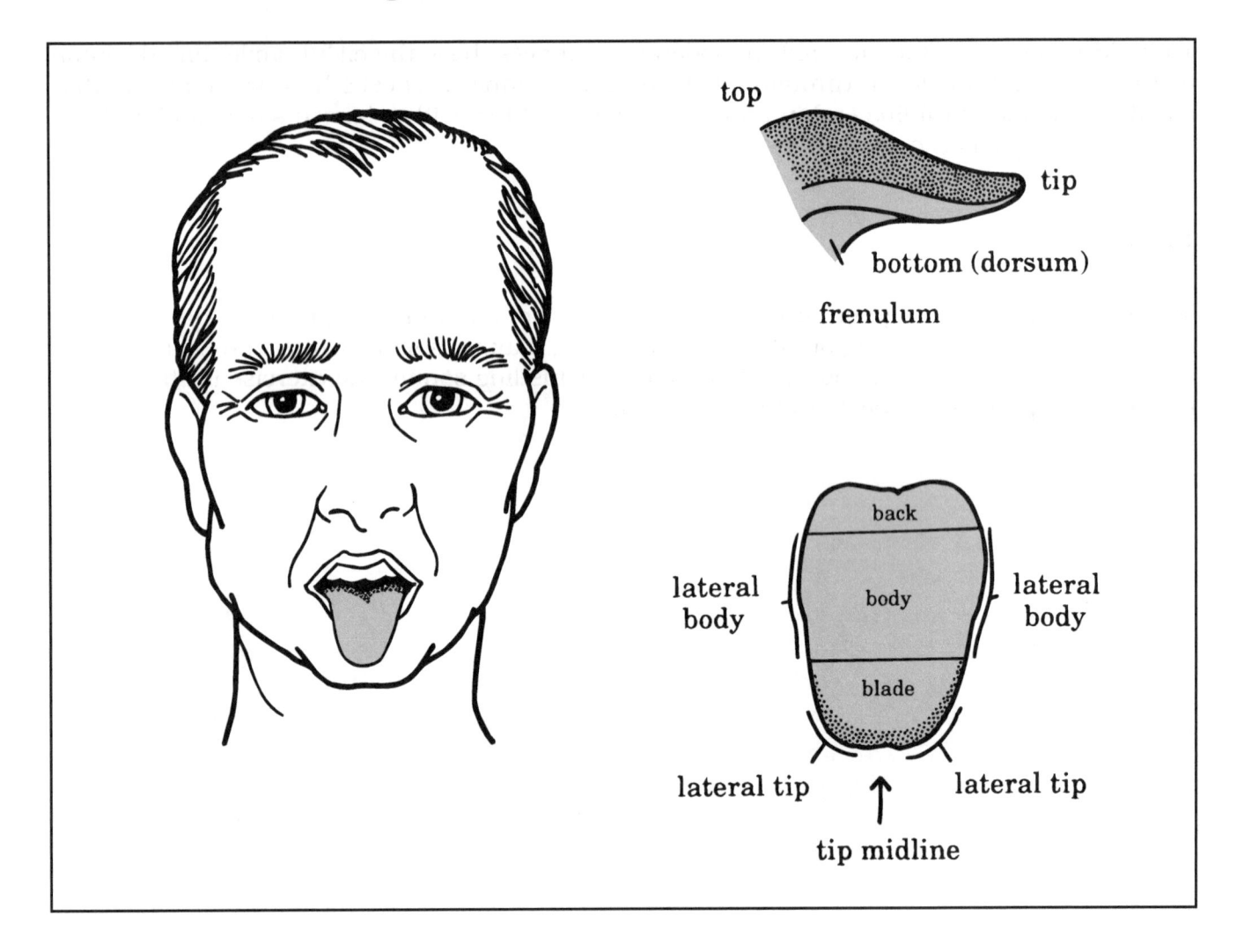

Protrude tongue downward toward chin with jaw open.

> Note: Use a mirror for this and all other tongue exercises for visual cues and reinforcement of proper positioning.

Benefits

- stretches and strengthens tongue
- improves range of motion anteriorly
- teaches parts of the tongue

Tongue and Inner Lip Massage

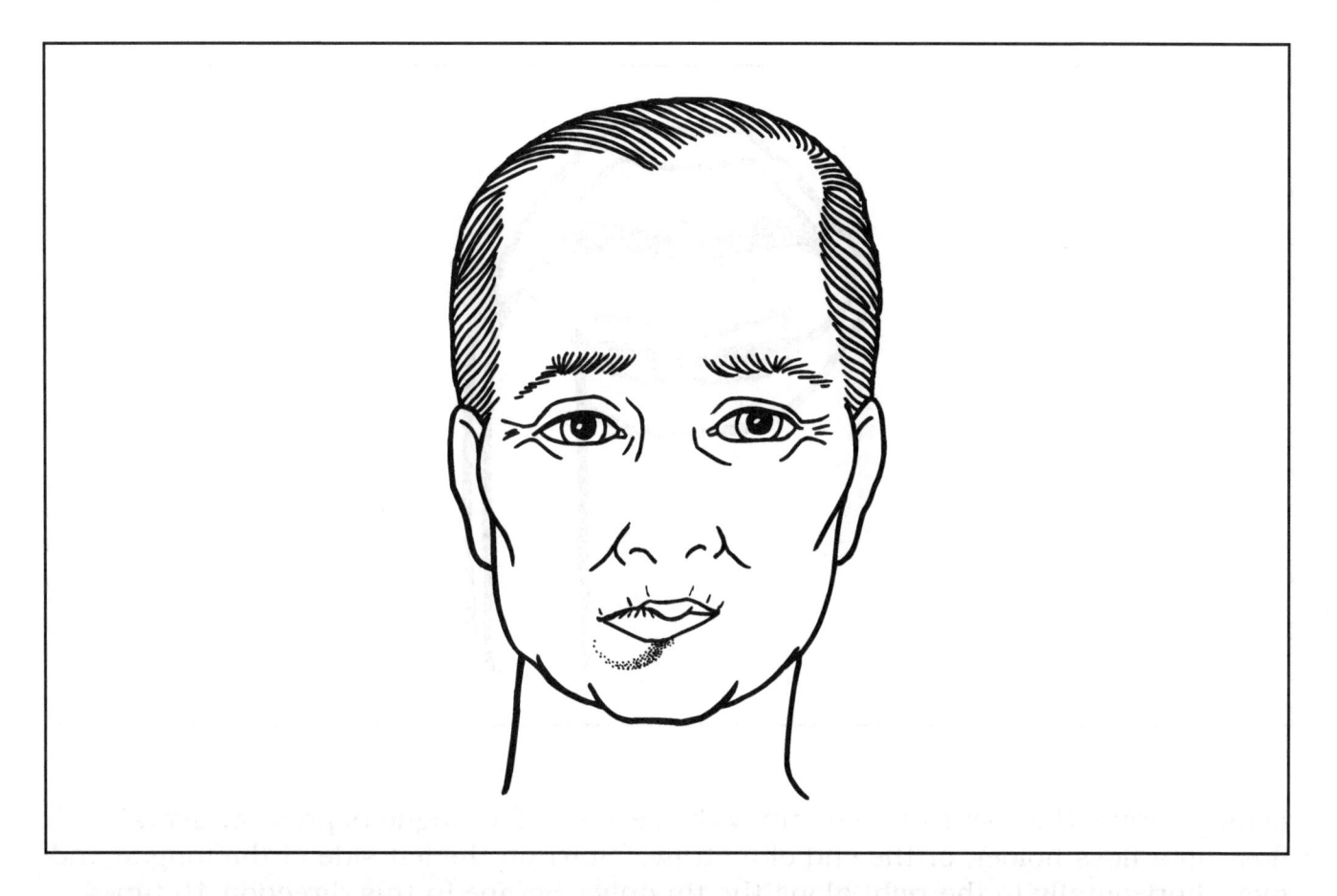

Chapter 11, *continued*

Push the inner lip out with the tongue. Press hard. Run it all around the lips, pushing hard. If the tongue is kept pushing forward around the lips, it will aim to strengthen the base and mid-sections of the tongue. It will also help to establish tongue tip control. Repeat around the lips 10 to 15 times.

To work the mid-sides of the tongue, widen the range of motion of the tongue to the sides of the cheeks. Continue in the same manner pushing the tongue into the cheek making a circular motion a few times. Then move to the other cheek. Remind the client to "push hard" and "let me see your tongue point out as if it is going to go through your cheek."

Benefits

- strengthens base and midsections of tongue
- improves tongue control

The Oral-Facial Therapy Exercise Book
2021 Edition

Tongue Tip Scrape

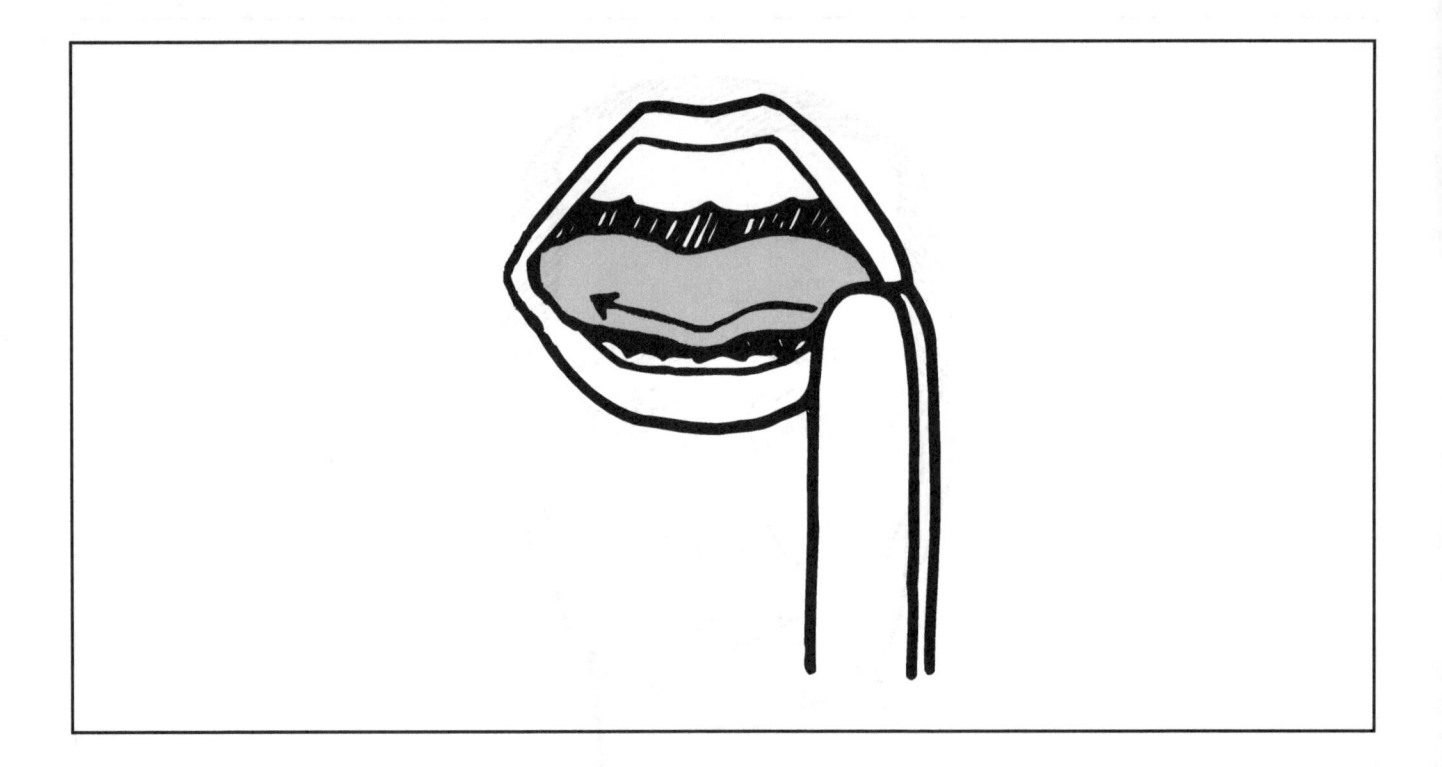

Chapter 11, continued

Lightly scrape the client's tongue tip with the edge of a tongue depressor, dental floss on a floss holder, or the end of a straw. Start on the left side of the tongue and move horizontally to the right along the tip only. Scrape in this direction 10 times. Then start on the right side and move along to the left along the tip only. Repeat 10 times in this direction.

Benefits

- widens tongue

- improves sensation awareness

- improves tip control

Tongue Click

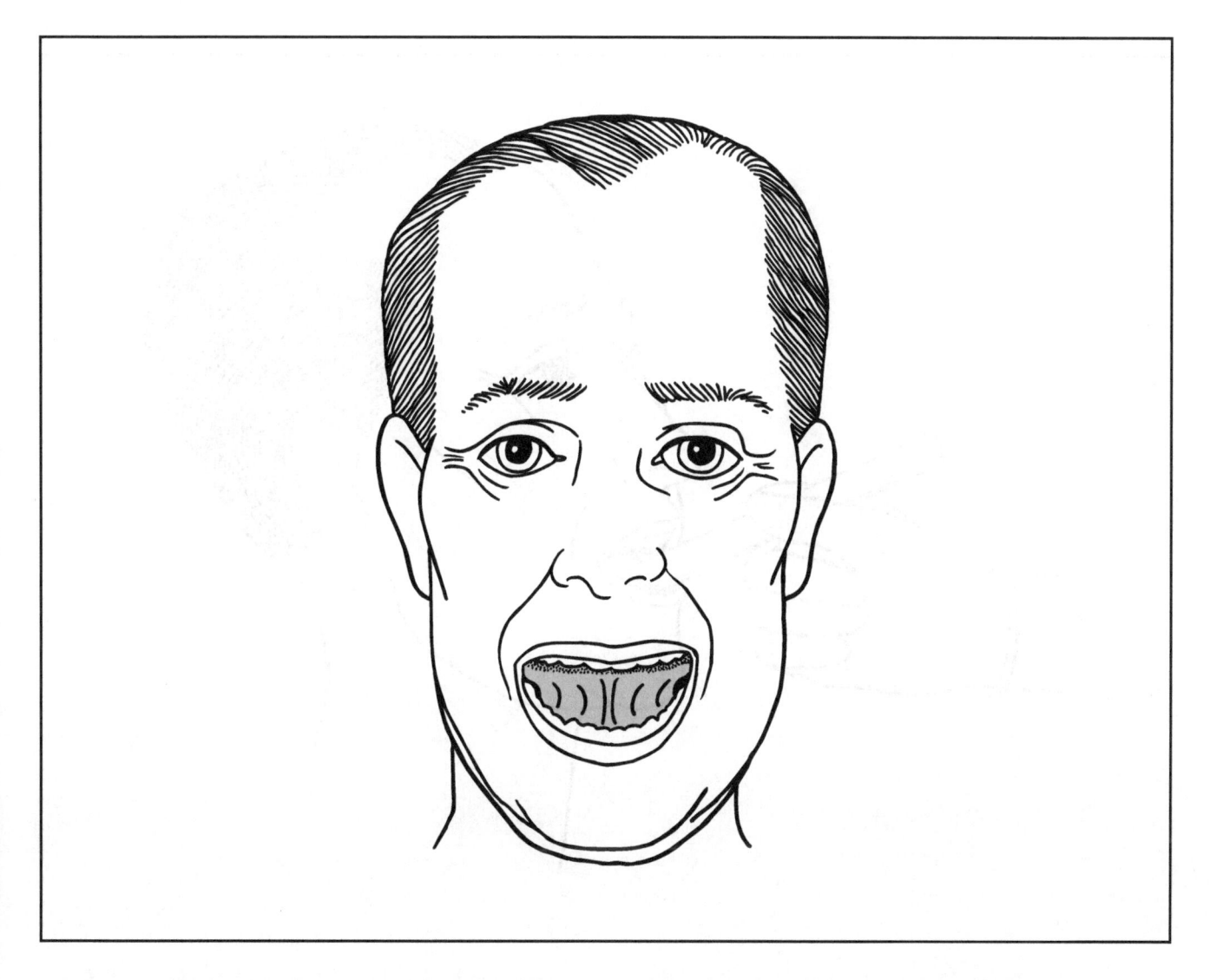

Chapter 11, continued

Click tongue against hard palate, making a loud clucking noise. Repeat for about 1 minute. Then click tongue with teeth clenched and jaw stabilized. Again, repeat for about 1 minute.

> Note: This exercise may be practiced with the tongue tip only for a tip strengthening exercise. The noise produced will be quieter but will help with forming the sucking action of the tongue.

Benefits

- improves medial tongue raise and tongue widening
- increases bolus retention and transit of bolus during swallowing

The Oral-Facial Therapy Exercise Book
2021 Edition

Tip Only Resistance

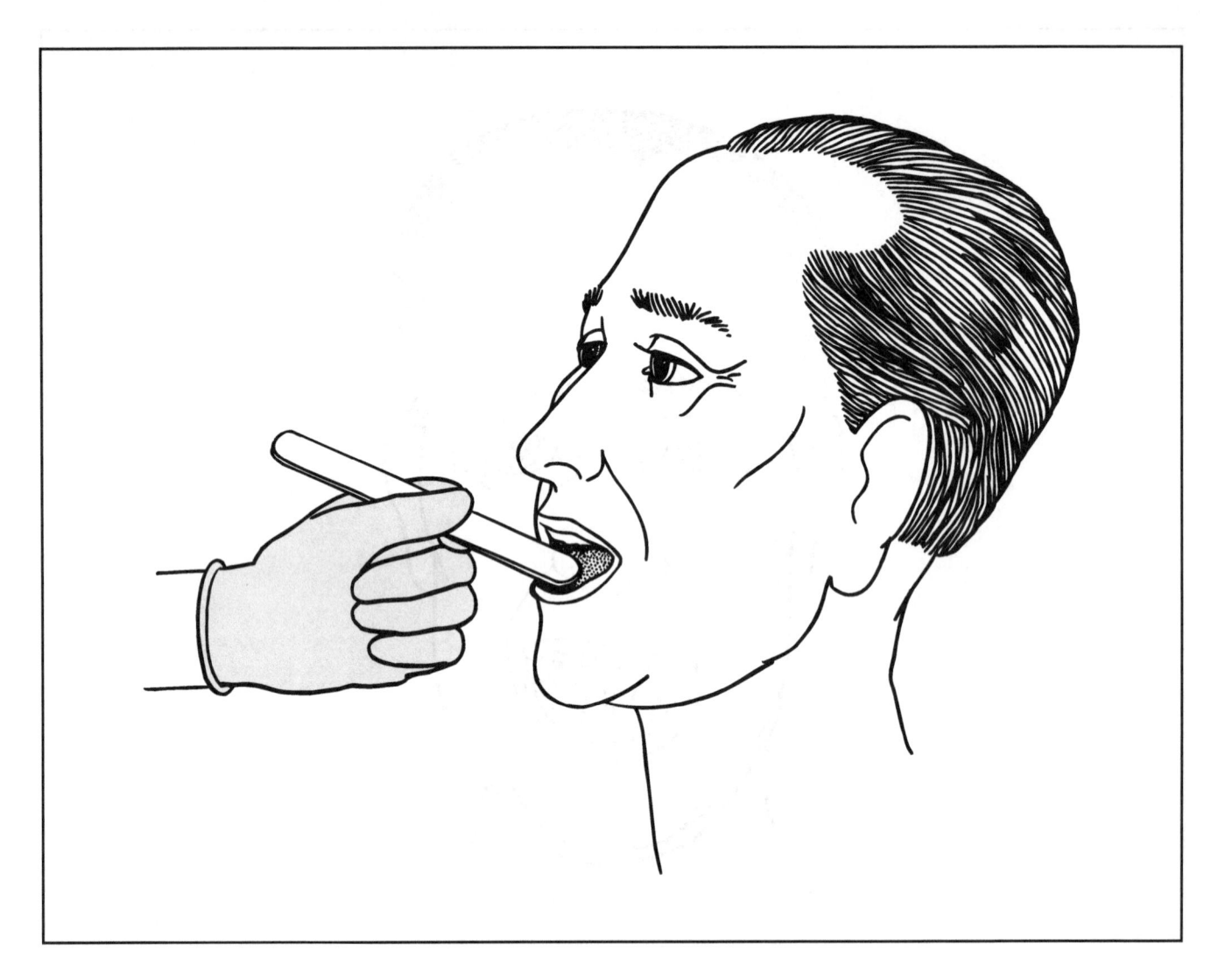

Chapter 11, continued

Apply and sustain downward pressure on the tongue tip only with the flat surface of a tongue depressor. Hold for 5 seconds. Repeat 3 to 5 times.

Note: Say "push up" to increase effort.

Benefit

- improves ability to raise tongue tip

Push Up to Bowl

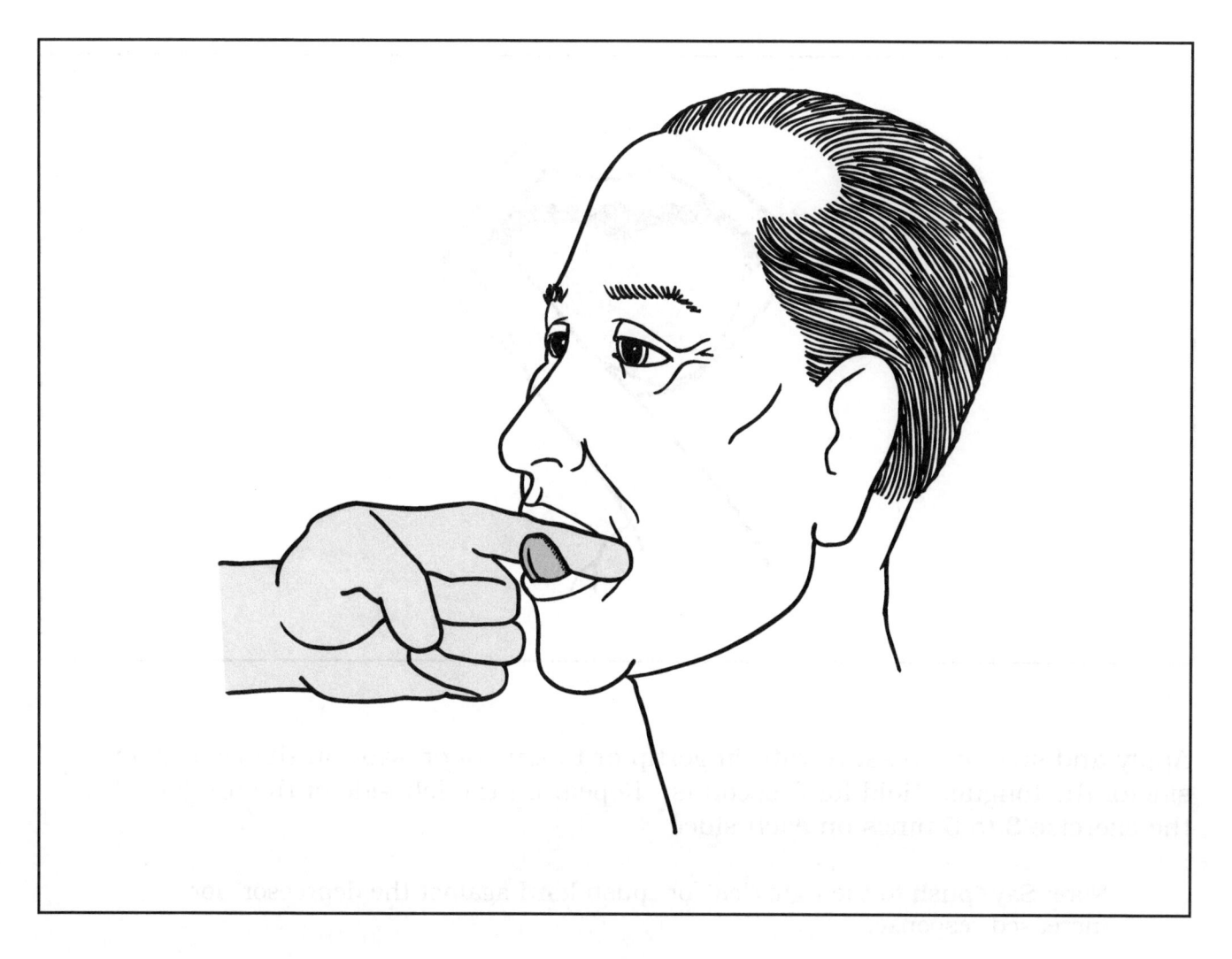

Chapter 11, *continued*

Apply and sustain slight downward pressure on the surface of the tongue blade with the side of index finger. Hold for 5 seconds. Resistance of the tongue will produce a bowl-like motion of the tongue needed to hold a bolus. Repeat 3 to 5 times.

  Note: Say "push up" to increase effort.

Benefits

○ increases bolus retention and transit of bolus during swallowing

○ strengthens tongue

Lateral Side Resistance

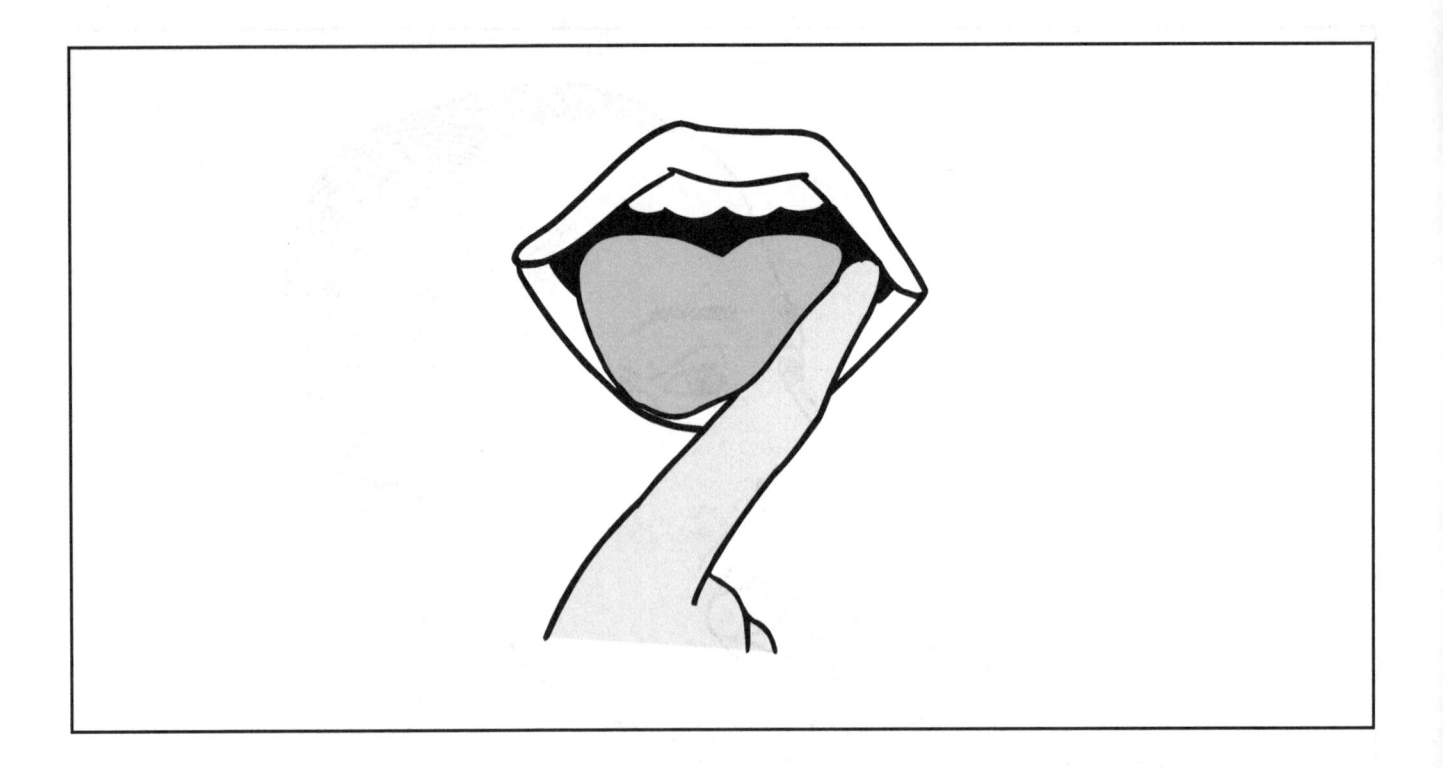

Chapter 11, continued

Apply and sustain pressure with fingertip or tongue depressor on the right (lateral) side of the tongue. Hold for 5 seconds. Repeat on the left side of the tongue. Do the exercise 3 to 5 times on each side.

> Note: Say "push to the right/left" or "push hard against the depressor" for increased response.

Benefit

- encourages lateral motion and opposite lateral raising of the tongue

Push Up to Flat Tongue

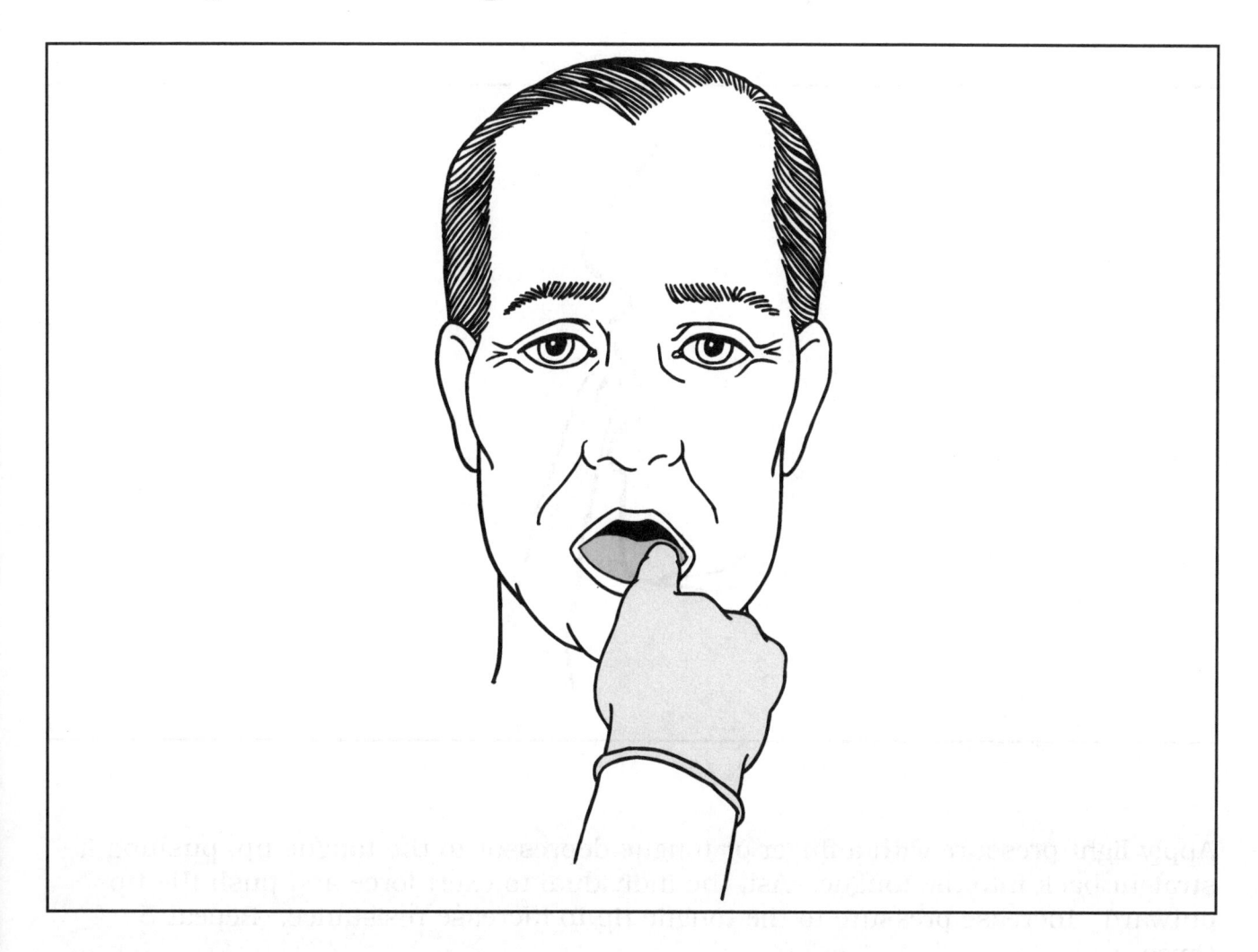

Chapter 11, continued

Apply pressure with a fingertip or tongue depressor flat on the top of the tongue <u>to the right of the midline</u> over the tip, blade, and body of the tongue. Avoid pressure to the back of the tongue. Hold for 5 seconds. Repeat on the left side. Do the exercise on each side.

Use a tongue depressor, Popsicle stick, or lollipop for resistance to the top surface of the tongue. Place the tongue depressor on the tongue and have the client push his tongue up against the tongue depressor. Encourage the client to hold the pressure for 1 to 5 seconds.

Benefit

- stimulates elevation of the body of the tongue

Blunted Tongue Tip Resistance

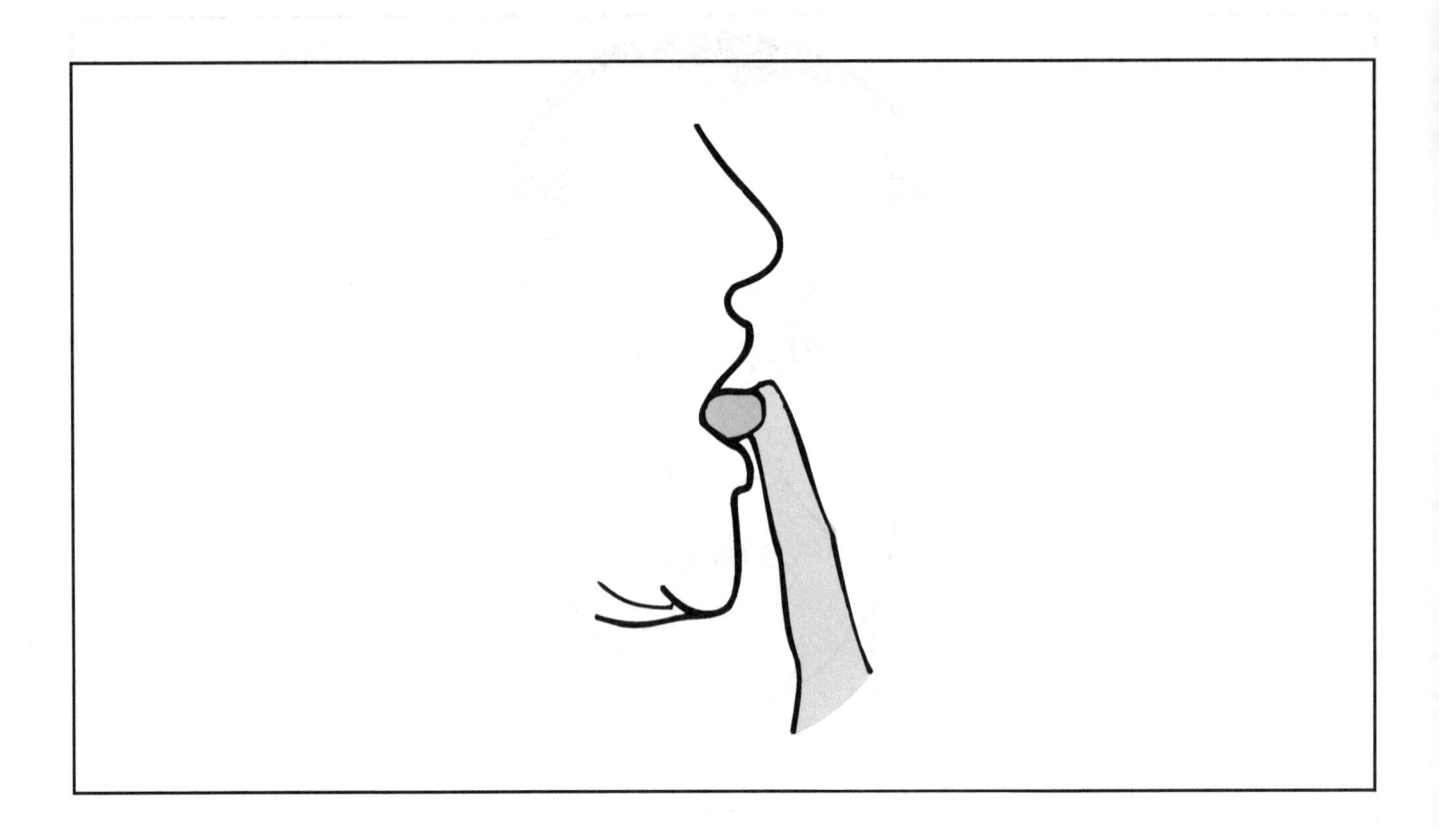

Chapter 11, continued

Apply light pressure with a finger or tongue depressor to the tongue tip, pushing it straight back into the tongue. Ask the individual to exert force and push the tip outward. Increase pressure to the tongue tip to increase resistance. Repeat 5 times.

Benefit

- strengthens and widens tongue

Brush Back Tip Curl Formation

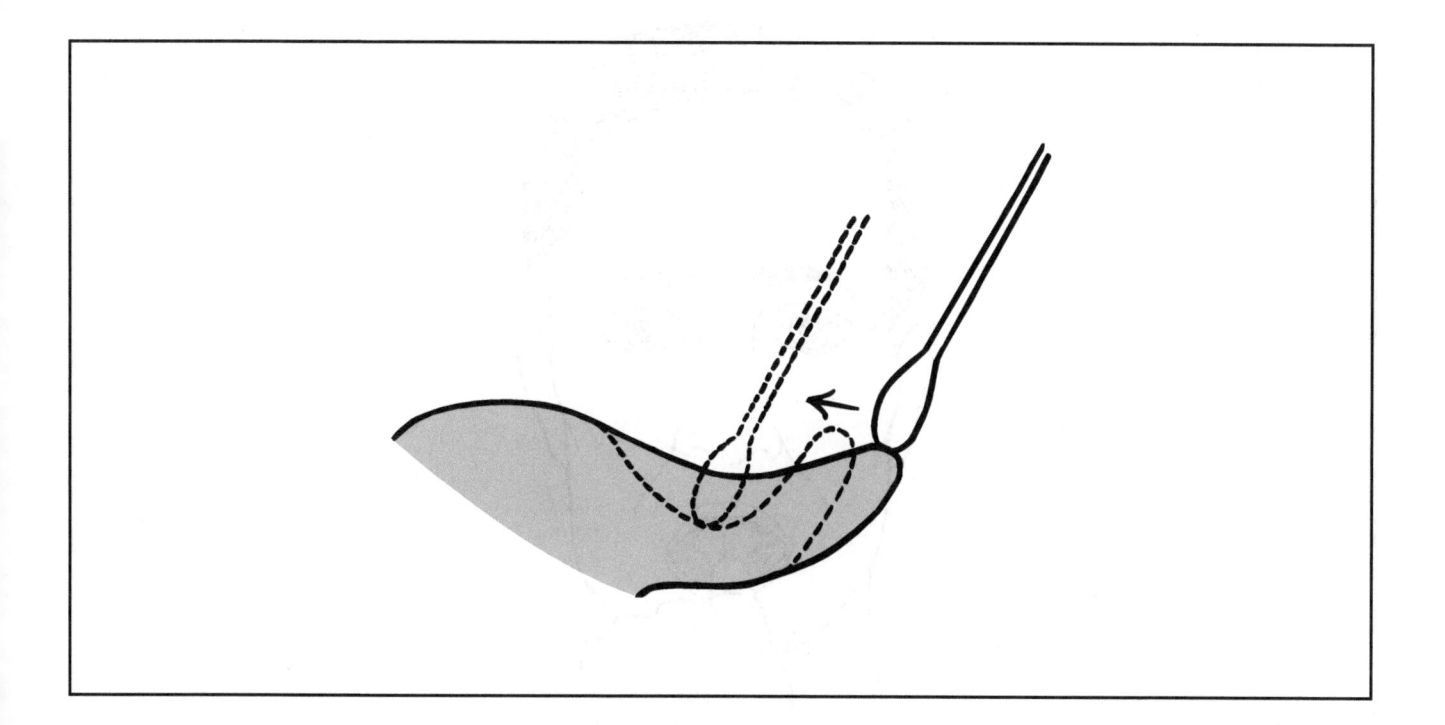

Chapter 11, *continued*

Start at the tip of the tongue at the midline and brush back approximately one inch on the blade of the tongue. The backward-only motion will stimulate an upward movement of the tongue tip. Repeat 10 times.

You can use a tongue depressor, gloved fingertip, or cotton-tip applicator.

Benefit

- assists in bolus formation

Tongue Frenulum Stretch

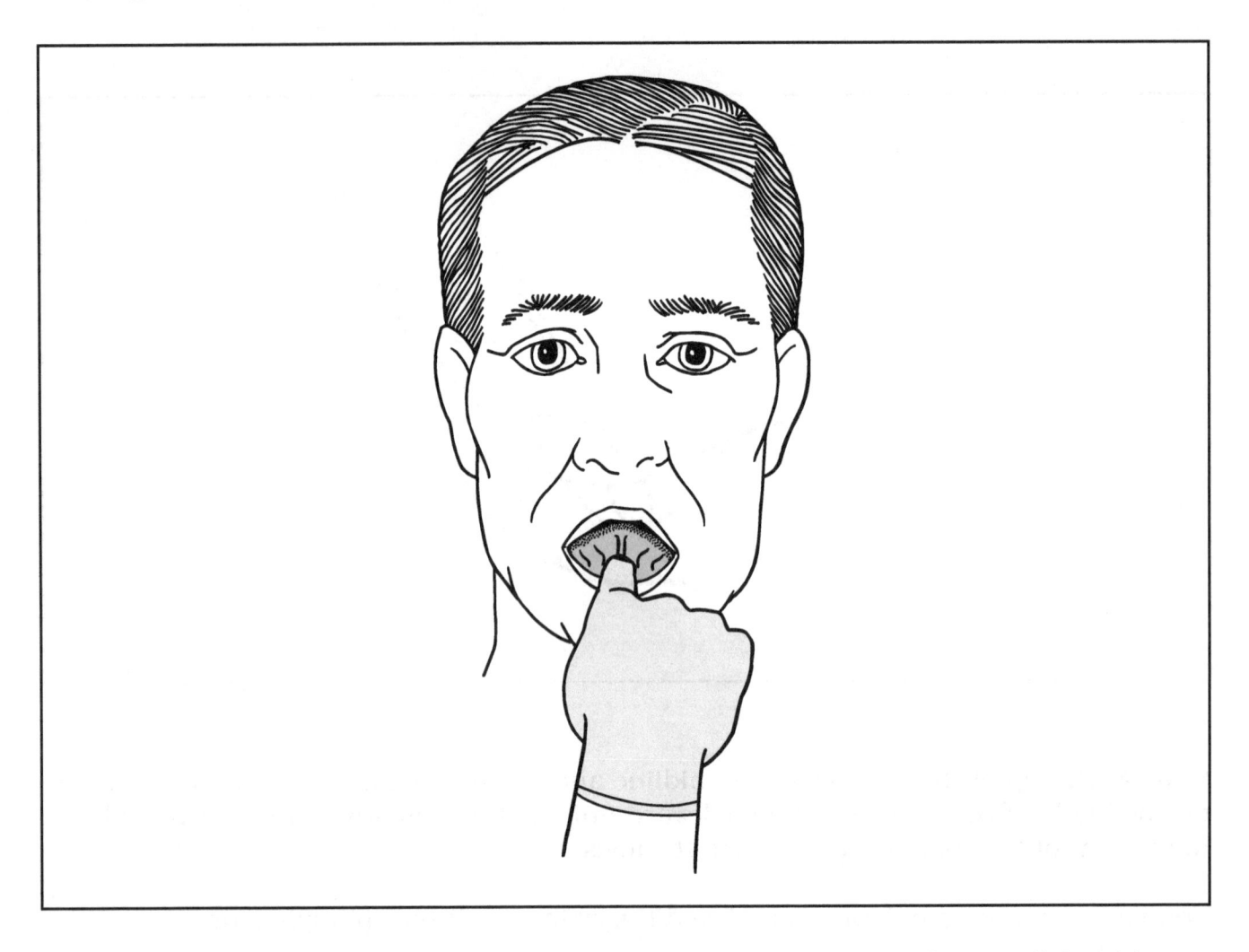

Chapter 11, continued

The tongue frenulum can restrict range of motion of the tongue for the /l/, /d/, /t/, and /th/ phonemes. When the tongue is restricted, it will form a heart and/or split down the middle when extended forward. In many cases, stretching the frenulum will reduce the need for surgery.

Have the individual open his mouth. Slide the flat side of your index finger under the tongue and apply light to moderate pressure against the stringy portion of the frenulum. Push straight back. Hold for 30 seconds. Repeat 3 times. Do this exercise 3 to 5 times a day. After facilitating this stretch for the client, show him how to place his finger on his frenulum for self-stretch practice.

Benefit

- increases range of motion of tongue

Tongue Widening

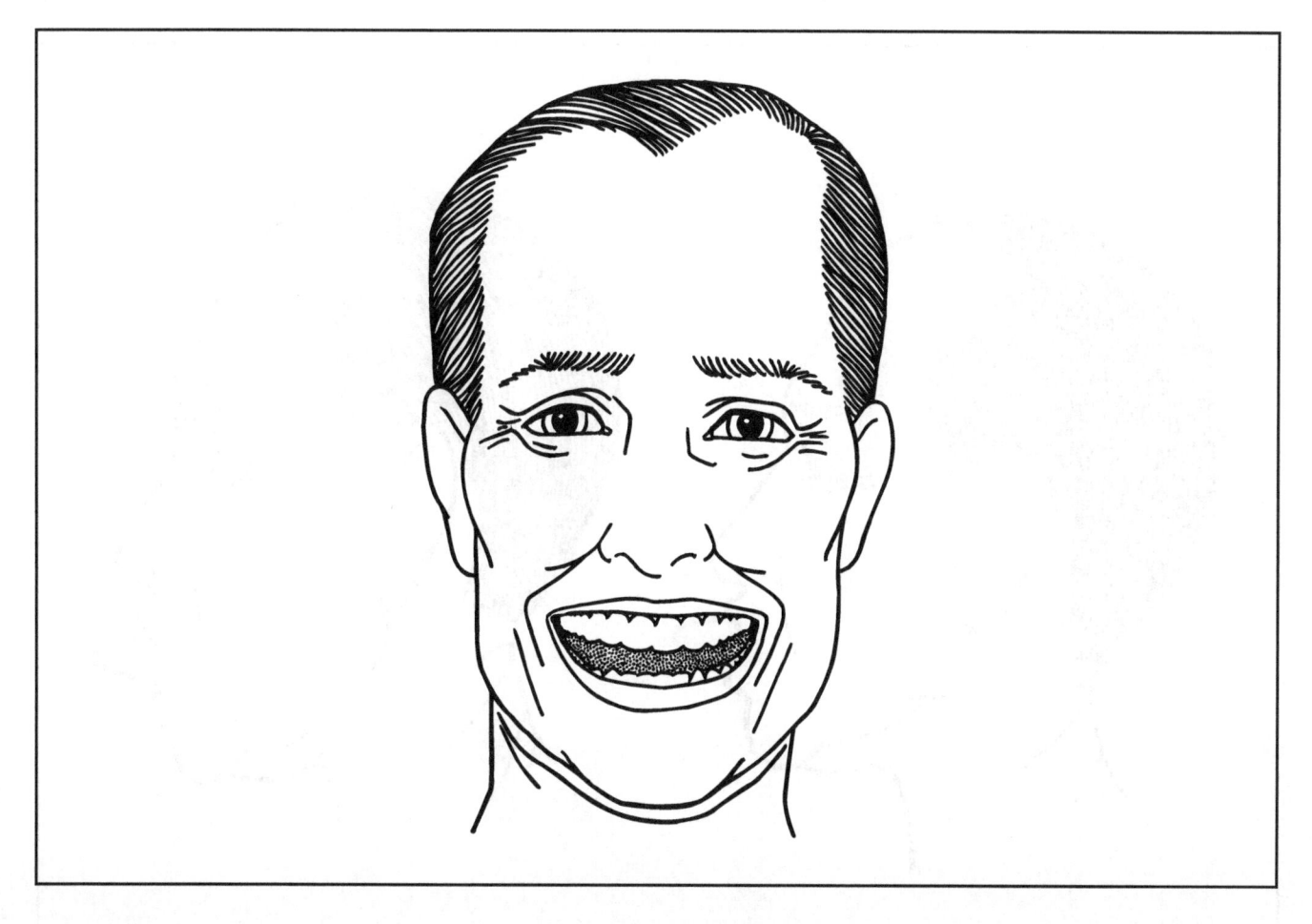

Chapter 11, continued

Have the individual say "ee" and elongate and exaggerate it. The tongue will widen naturally. Provide a model if necessary. It is best not to ask the individual to widen the tongue or to bring attention to the widening until he is able to establish it by practicing the "ee" sound.

While the client is holding the "ee" sound, show him how the tongue touches the sides of his teeth. Ask him to hold it there after the "ee" sound is finished. Eventually the client should be able to widen his tongue voluntarily.

If the client's tongue gets tired or he forgets how to widen his tongue, have him produce an "ee" to retrain his tongue.

Benefits

- aids in correction of lateral lisping

Straight Tongue Stretch

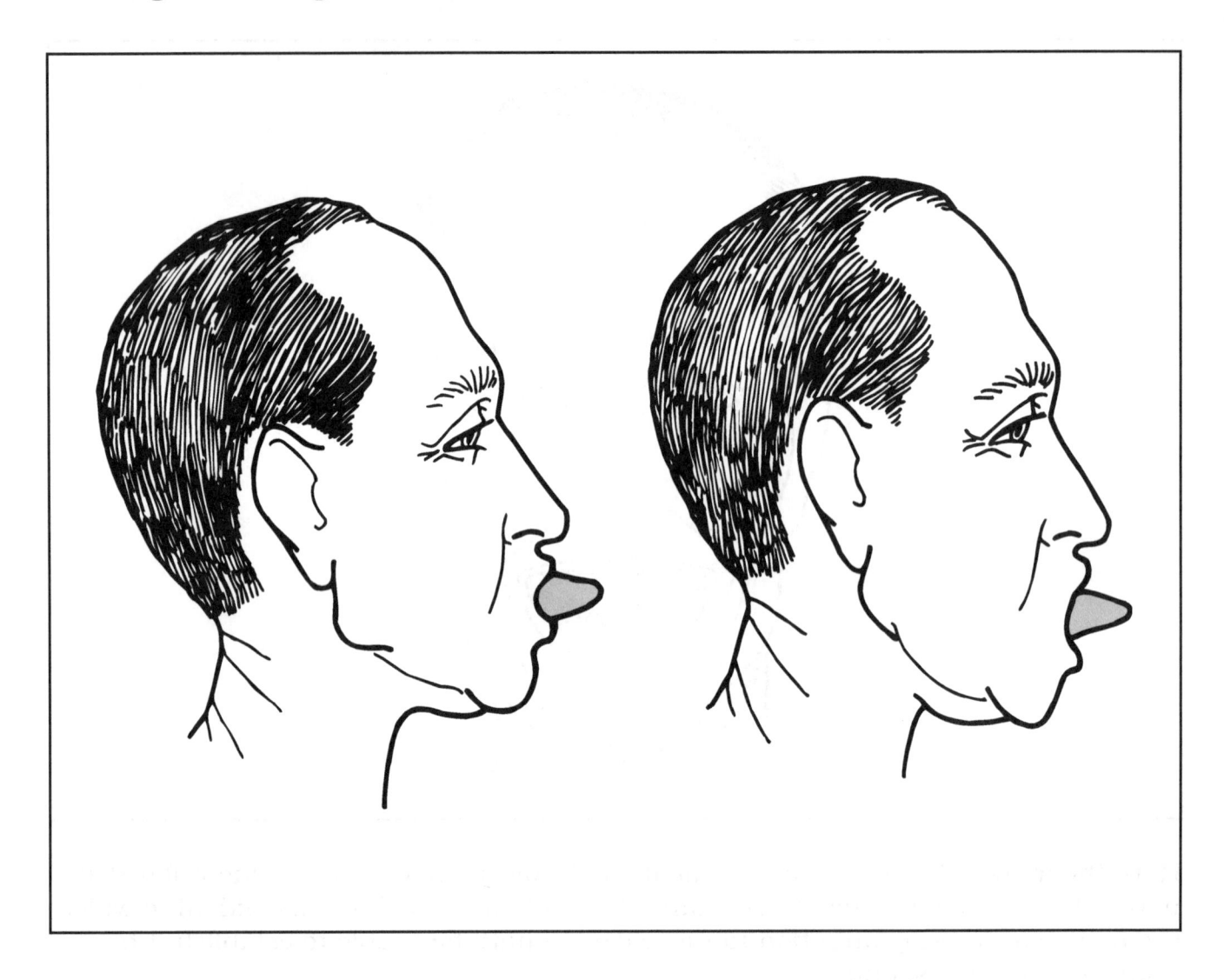

Chapter 11, continued

Stick tongue straight out as far as it will go with the mouth slightly open. Use full force when extending tongue.

Then stick the tongue straight out with the jaw open as wide as it will go. Hold tongue to full extension to stretch the bottom and back of tongue.

Benefit

- improves tongue extension and range of motion anteriorly

Tongue Tip Movement

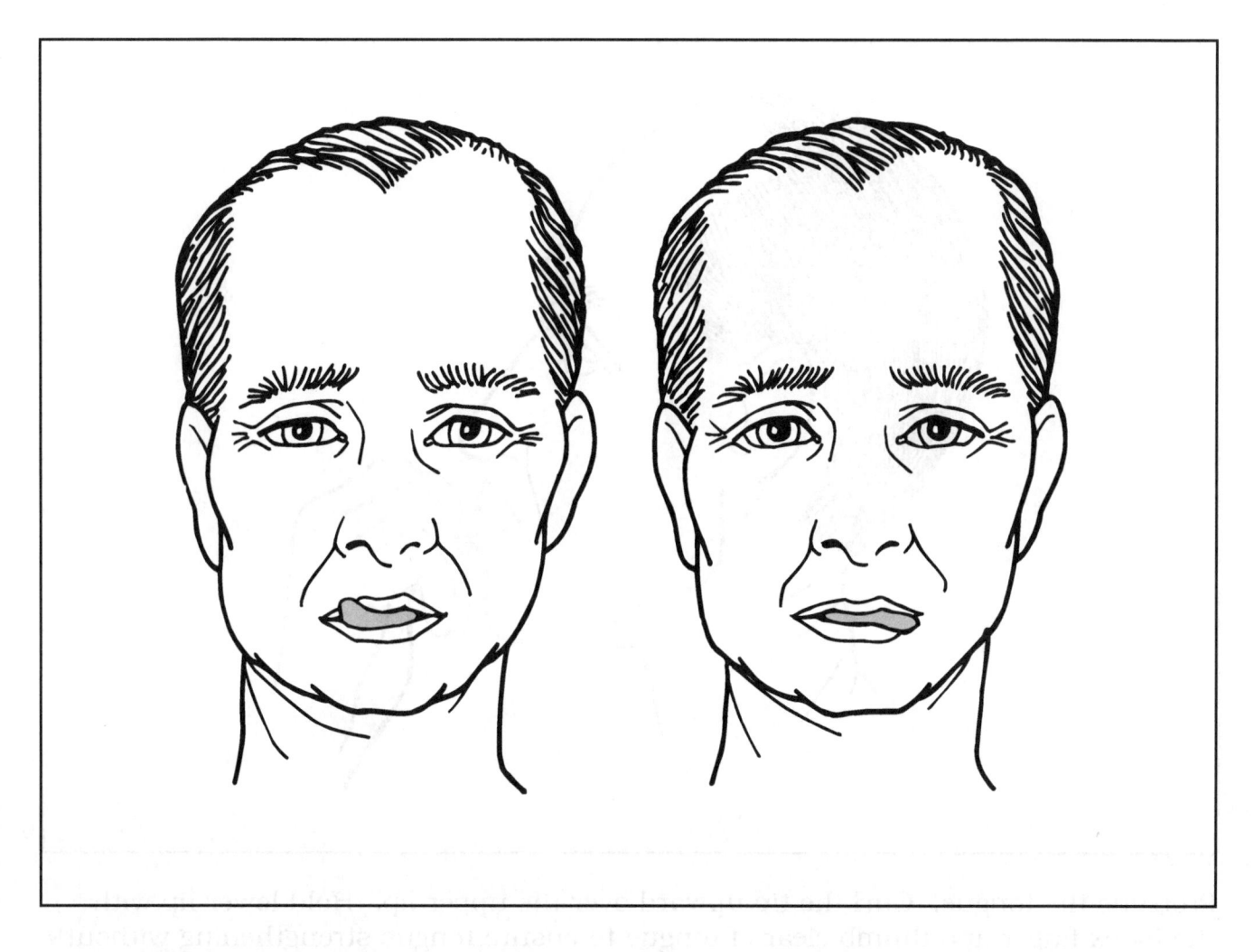

Chapter 11, continued

Protrude the tongue. Raise and lower the tongue as you lick your lips. Repeat. Gently bite on the blade of tongue to allow tongue tip movement only. If it helps, hold the lower lip down to ensure tongue tip movement only.

Benefit

○ improves tongue tip awareness, agility, strength, and range of motion

Upper Tongue Tip Raise

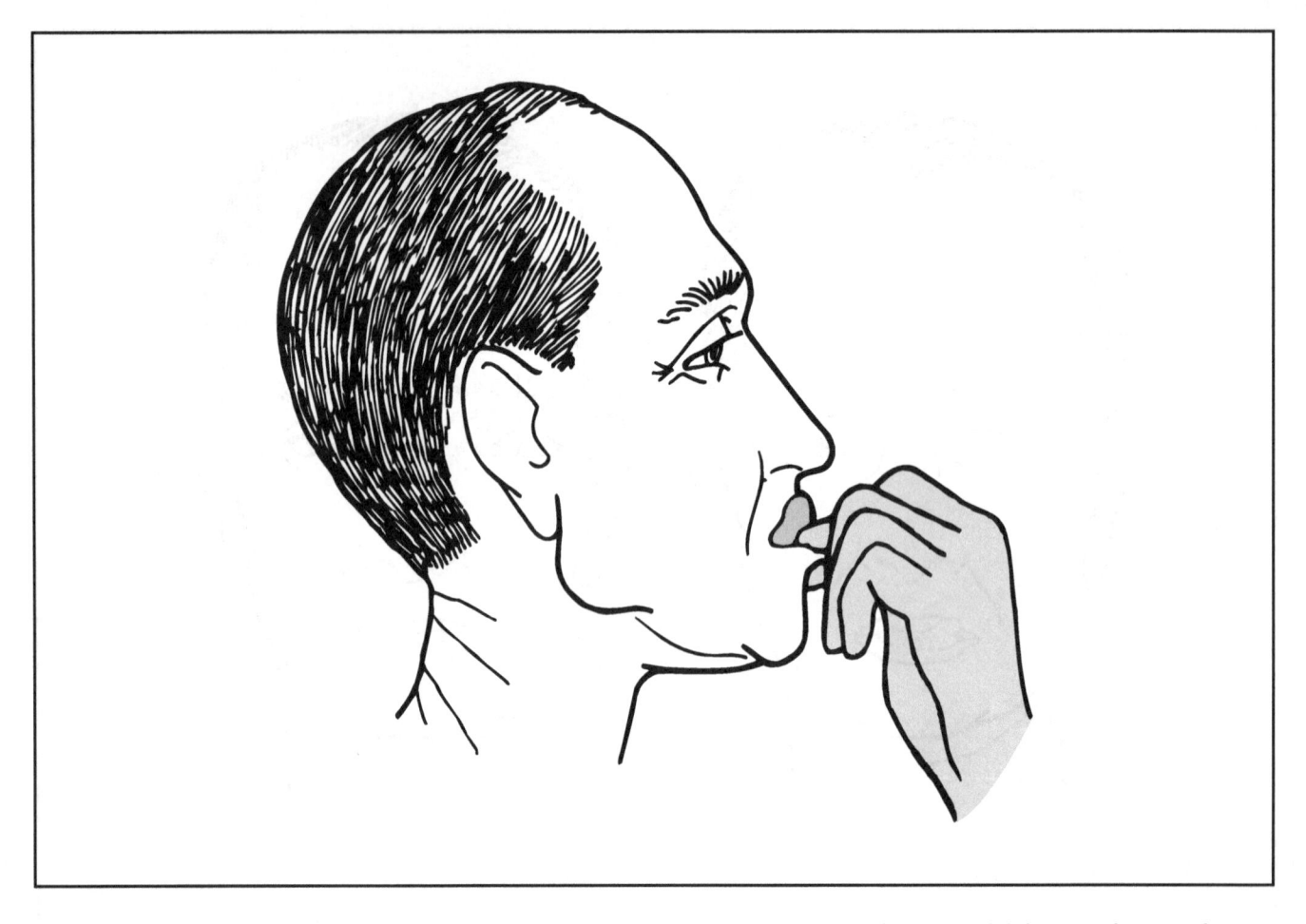

Chapter 11, continued

Protrude the tongue. Curl the tip upward over the upper lip. Hold lower lip with the index finger and thumb clear of tongue to ensure tongue strengthening without lower lip assist. Gently bite on mid-portion of the tongue to isolate tip raising and increase complexity.

Try curling the tip up with a skinny tongue and then a wide tongue.

    Note: Use a mirror to improve accuracy.

Benefits

- stretches and strengthens tongue raise
- improves range of motion anteriorly
- assists in pre-speech formation of /th, l, t, d/

Tongue Tip Raise

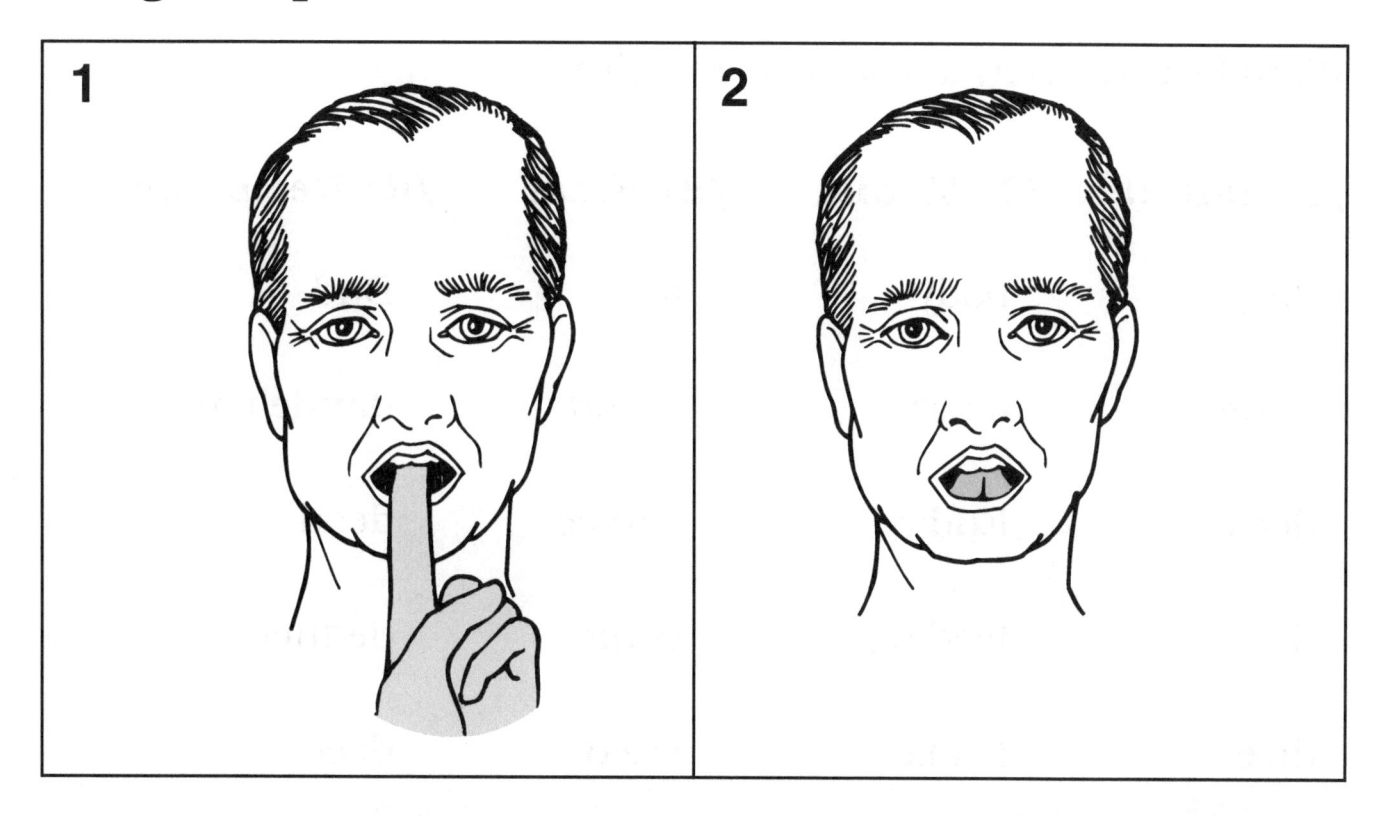

Chapter 11, continued

Place a finger on the gum ridge behind the upper front teeth as shown in picture 1. Touch the tip of the tongue to this spot as shown in picture 2.

Hold the tip of the tongue to the spot for at least five seconds. Increase time to 30 seconds, continuing to press tip onto the spot.

Touch the tongue tip to the spot and say, "tee . . . tee . . . tee . . . tee . . ."
"lee . . . lee . . . lee . . . lee . . ."
"dit . . . dit . . . dit . . . dit . . ."

Exercises listed for tongue tip raise and articulation practice of the sounds /t, l, d/ in words and sentences.

Benefit

- strengthens tongue tip

Word Lists for *Tongue Tip Raise* Exercise

/d/ Initial	/d/ Medial	/d/ Final	/d/ Recurring
deep	body	add	Dad
dance	cider	bread	dandelion
deck	Eddie	carved	dead
dish	feeding	could	deduction
dive	Friday	cried	deed
do	hiding	made	defend
doll	Judy	fed	did
done	lady	food	disorder
duke	pudding	good	dived
dump	soda	head	Donald
dinner	today	lemonade	doodle
dizzy	wedding	salad	dude

Chapter 11, continued

Word Lists for *Tongue Tip Raise* Exercise

/l/ Initial	/l/ Medial	/l/ Final	/l/ Recurring
lamp	alarm	April	label
land	alike	cool	lamplight
lawn	allow	female	landlady
leap	ballet	goal	legal
learn	believe	meatball	lifeline
leg	belong	pale	lilac
leaf	caller	pool	local
lick	color	seashell	loll
limp	Dallas	toenail	lollipop
load	fallen	towel	lonely
look	gallon	wall	loyal
love	Jell-O	yell	skillfully

The Oral-Facial Therapy Exercise Book
2021 Edition

Chapter 11, continued

Word Lists for *Tongue Tip Raise* Exercise

/t/ Initial	/t/ Medial	/t/ Final	/t/ Recurring
taco	biting	about	saltwater
tail	city	basket	tablet
tea	cotton	closet	tasty
teacher	daughter	doormat	tattoo
ten	detail	forget	taught
tiger	eating	meat	tight
tiny	fatter	pat	toaster
toe	heater	wet	tomato
took	hotter	nut	tot
toy	kitten	ate	total
tuna	petal	bite	turtle
turkey	sweeter	feet	tutor

The Oral-Facial Therapy Exercise Book
2021 Edition

Chapter 11, continued

Sentences for *Tongue Tip Raise* Exercise

1. Let's have tea instead of coffee.
2. My daughter lives in Colorado.
3. He taught me how to make tacos Friday.
4. We love to eat lime Jell-O.
5. I saw the ballet in Dallas.
6. April is a good month to go to European cities.
7. Should I order cider or lemonade?
8. She collects dishes, dolls, and seashells.
9. Donald forgot to turn the heater down.
10. Pat brought me a lilac today.
11. The lawn is full of dandelions.
12. Eddie doodles turtles and kittens.
13. I like my cookies sweeter.
14. The teacher skillfully handled the debate.
15. The leaves have fallen early this year.
16. Donna adds bread to her meatballs.
17. Please give me a soda with dinner.
18. The groom felt dizzy before the wedding.
19. Do you get a tax deduction this year?
20. Helen carved the turkey for Judy.

Posterior Tongue Tip Sweep

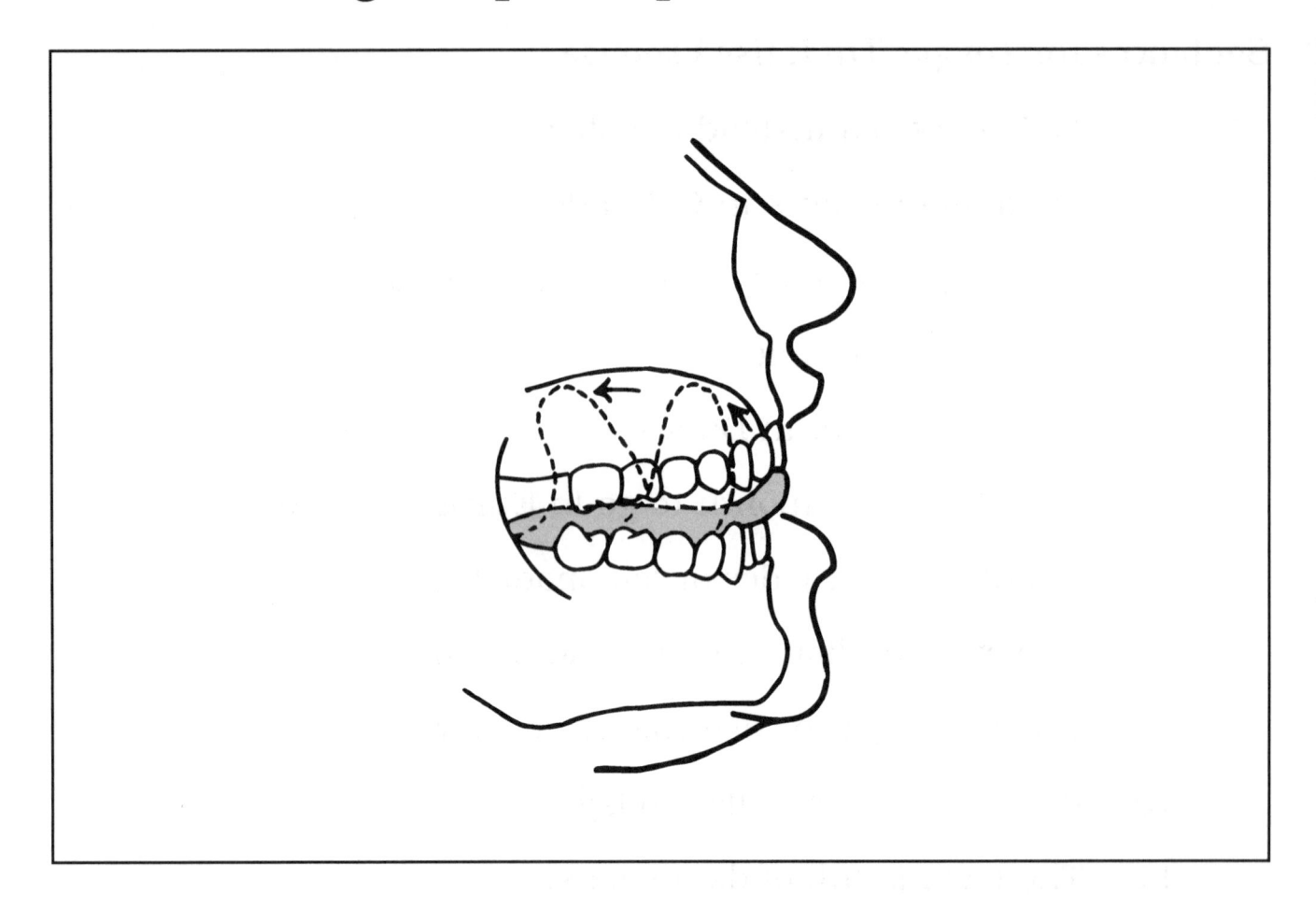

Chapter 11, continued

Touch tongue tip on the bottom of the upper front teeth. Slide tongue tip directly back along the roof of the mouth to the soft palate. Be sure to always touch the roof of the mouth. Stretch the tongue backward to full extension.

Practice with a skinny tongue using the tongue tip only. Then practice with a flat, wide tongue tip.

Benefits

- stretches and strengthens the tongue tip for improved range of motion for raising and retraction of the tongue

- assists in the formation of /l/ and /r/

- assists in bolus formation

Lateral Cheek/Tongue Sweep

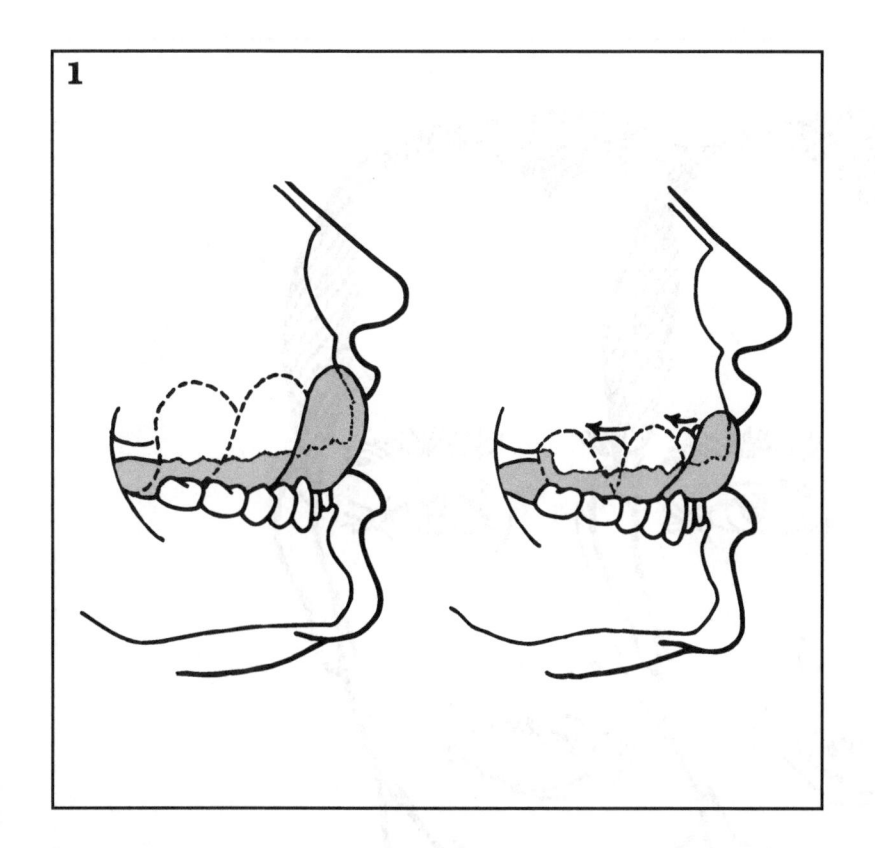

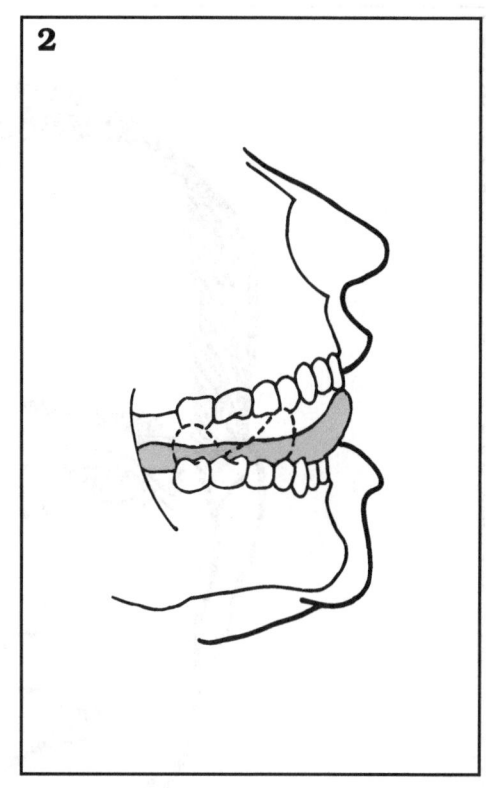

Chapter 11, *continued*

1. Place the tip of the tongue on the inside of the upper lip. Apply pressure to the tongue tip and move the tongue along the inner upper cheek all the way back to the right as shown in picture 1. Bring the tongue back along the inner cheek around to the left side. Repeat on the lower lip and cheek.

2. For more practice, move the tongue tip along the lower surface of the teeth all the way back to the last tooth on the right as shown in picture 2. Return using full motion as you glide the tongue tip to the last tooth on the left.

Benefits

- stretches and strengthens the tongue
- improves and increases range of motion
- assists in buccal (inner cheek) clearing

Lateral Tongue Stretch

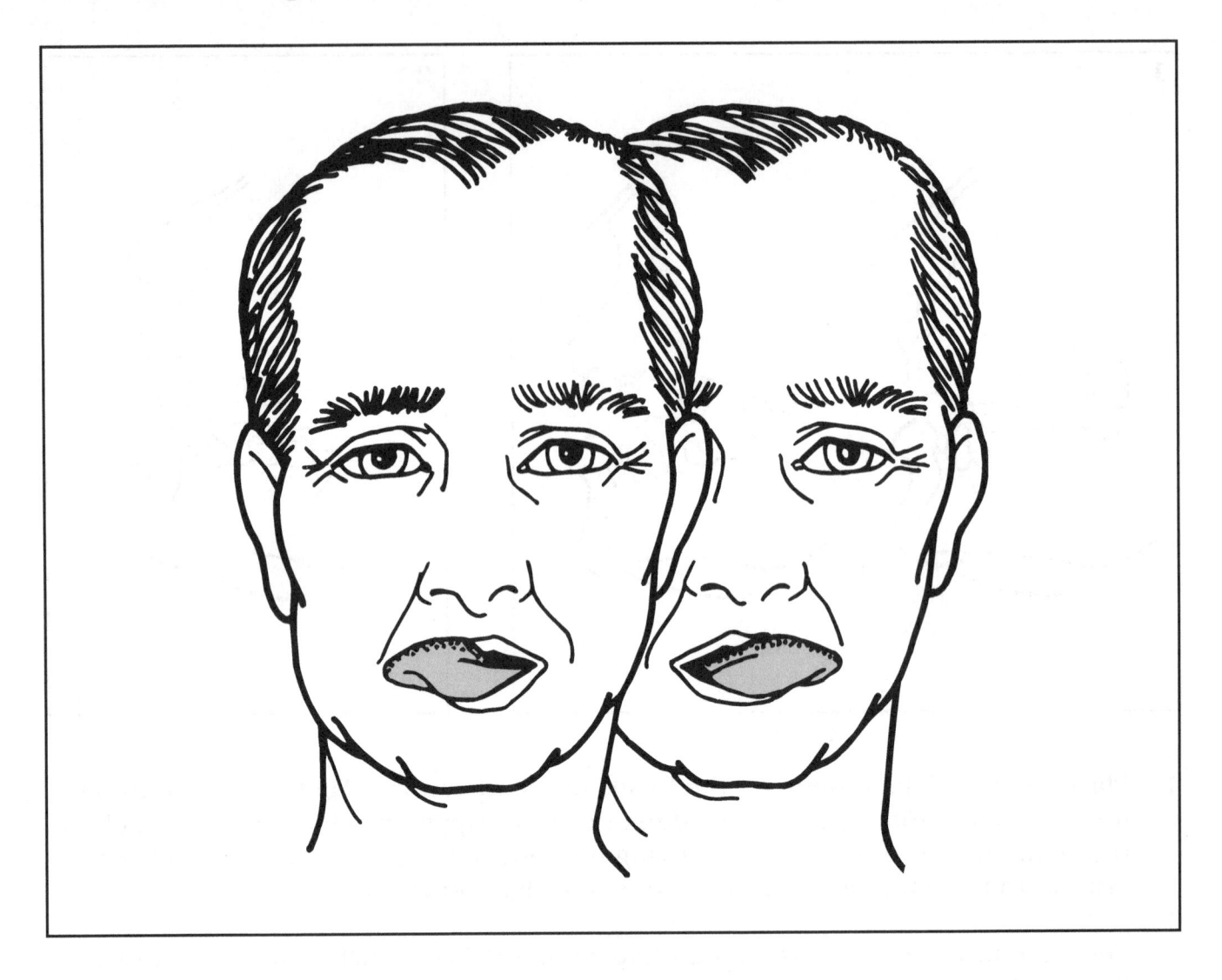

Chapter 11, *continued*

Protrude tongue to the right corner of the mouth. Hold to far right corner for 10 seconds. Switch to left corner of mouth, protruding tongue to full extension on the left side. Hold for 10 seconds.

For more practice, do the exercise with the jaw open wide.

Benefits

○ stretches and strengthens the back and lateral portions of the tongue

○ improves range of motion anteriorly

The Oral-Facial Therapy Exercise Book
2021 Edition

Chapter 12: Nasal Exercises

Sinus-Nasal Pressure Point Release

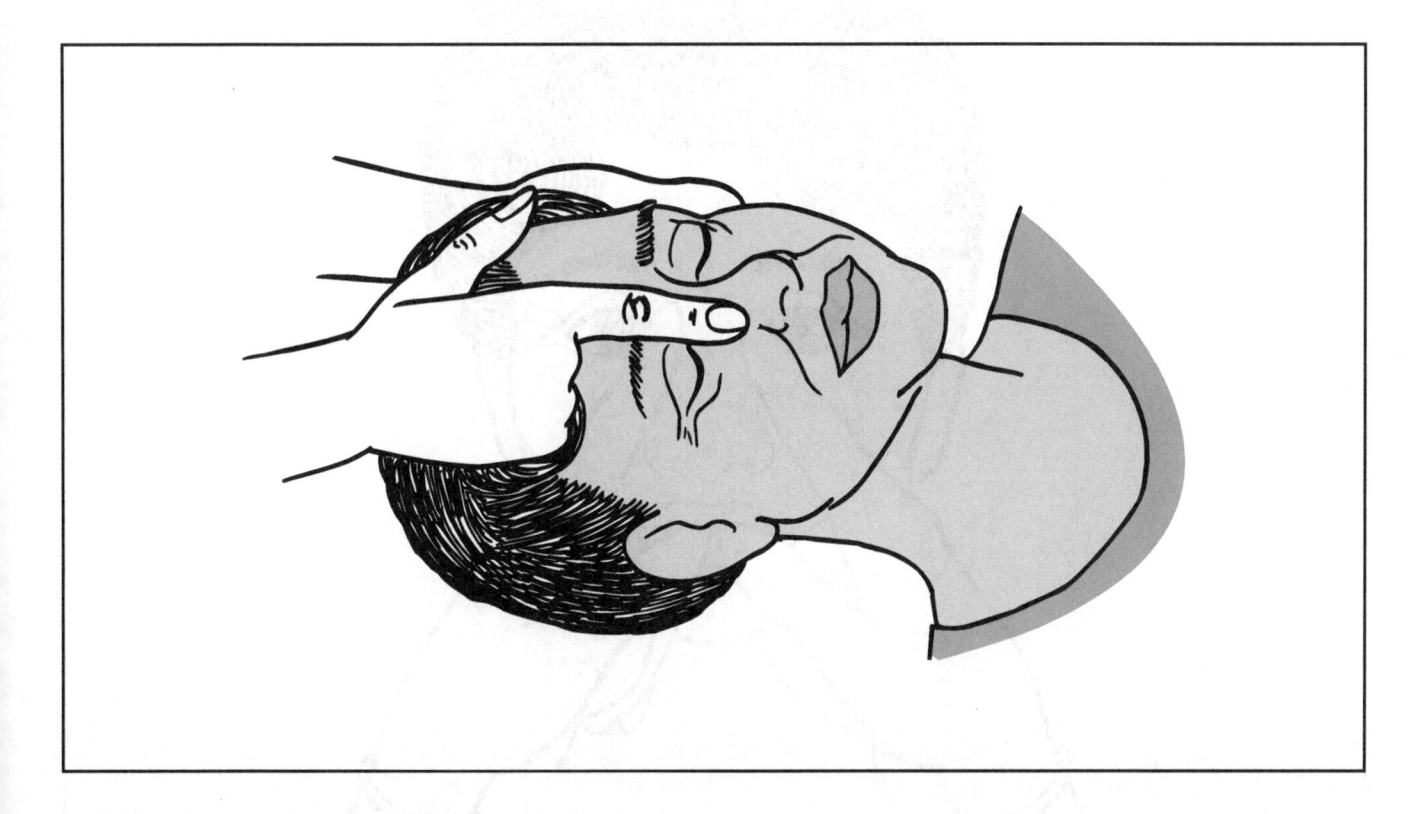

Hold the head with one hand and press against the side of the nose at adjacent spots from top to bottom with the other hand. Hold for 5 seconds at each spot. If you encounter a trigger point or place of muscle tension or discomfort, massage it in a little circle. Repeat on the other side.

To further stretch the muscles, extend fingers laterally down toward the cheek on each side of the nose. Keep finger placement on nose and avoid all contact of the eyes.

Benefit

- helps clear sinuses

Nasal Pressure

Chapter 12, continued

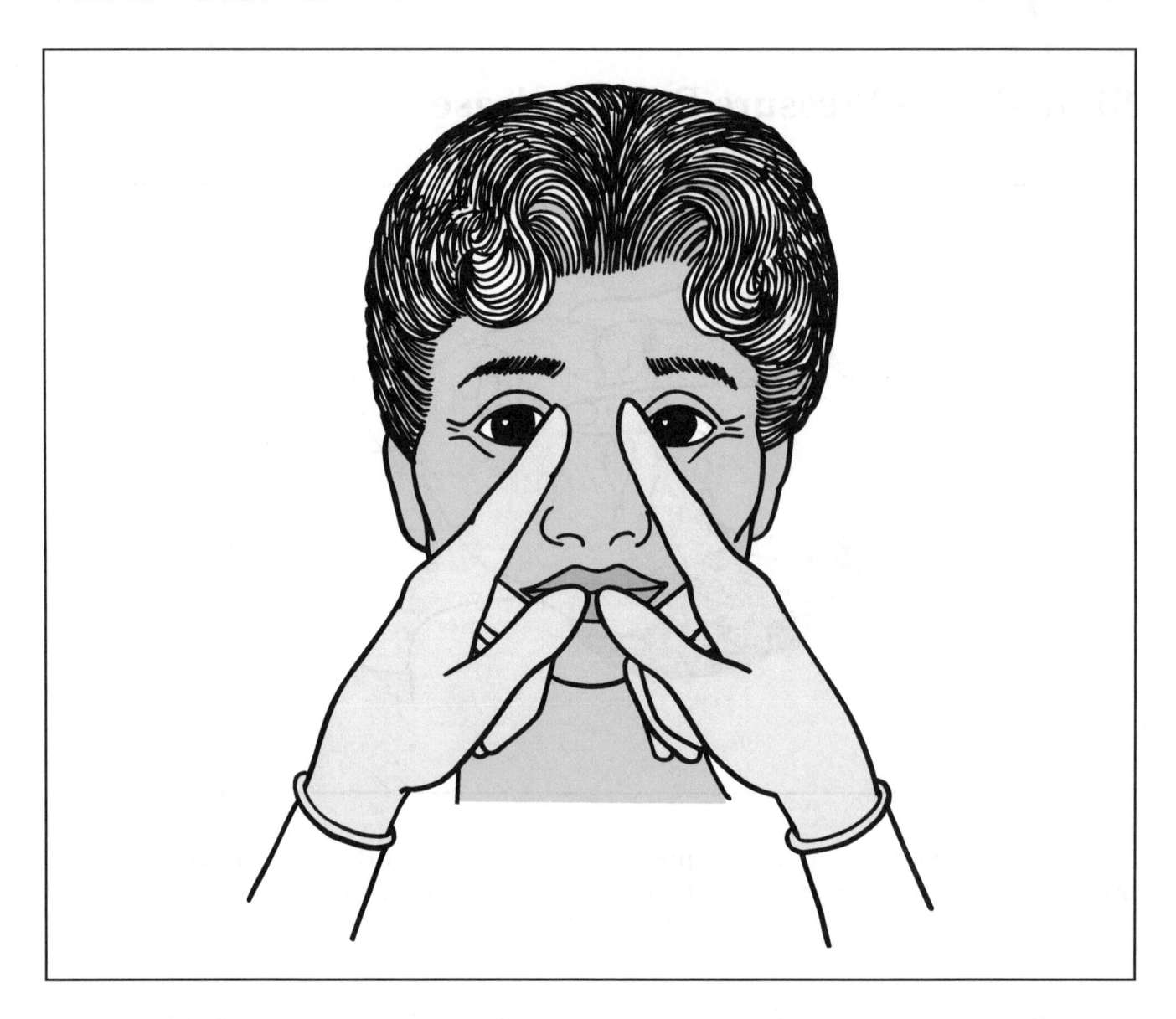

Use index fingers from each hand or use one hand in a "V" position. Apply pressure in toward the nose with fingers directly on either side of bridge of nose, slightly below eyebrows. Apply steady pressure, holding 10 to 15 seconds. Rest. Reapply pressure. Maintain relaxed brow, face, lips, neck, and jaw. Rest elbows on table for increased resistance. Keep finger placement on nose and avoid all contact with the eyes.

Benefits

- reduces eye muscle strain

- reduces headache and sinus pain

Nasal Pinch 1

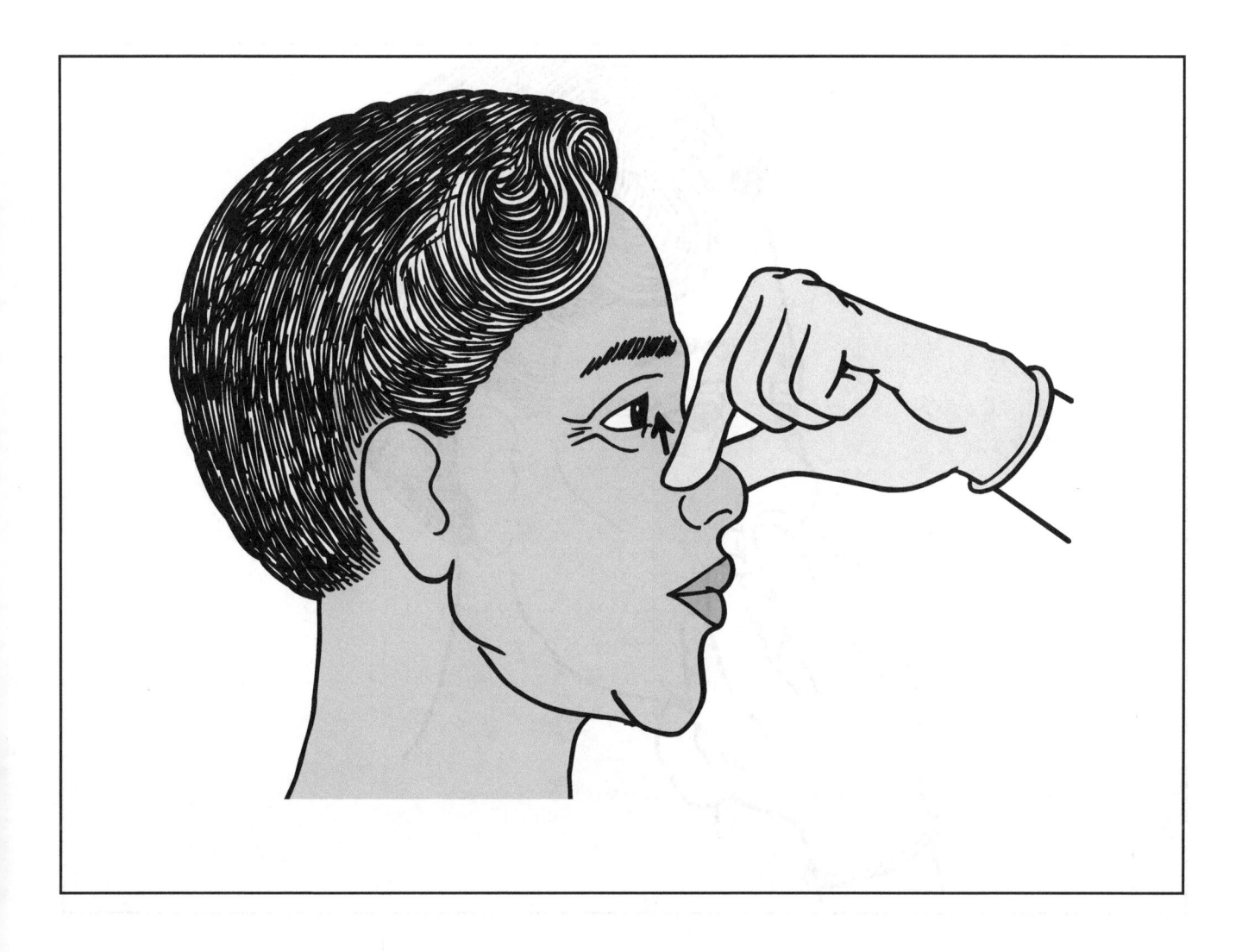

Chapter 12, *continued*

Apply pressure and pinch bridge of nose with thumb and forefinger. Squeeze and pull muscle upward and inward until fingers touch. Maintain relaxed brow, cheeks, neck, and jaw. Release after 10 to 15 seconds. Rest. Repeat.

Benefits

- reduces muscle tightness and strain associated with eyes and nose
- reduces facial strain and pain associated with sinus problems

Nasal Pinch 2

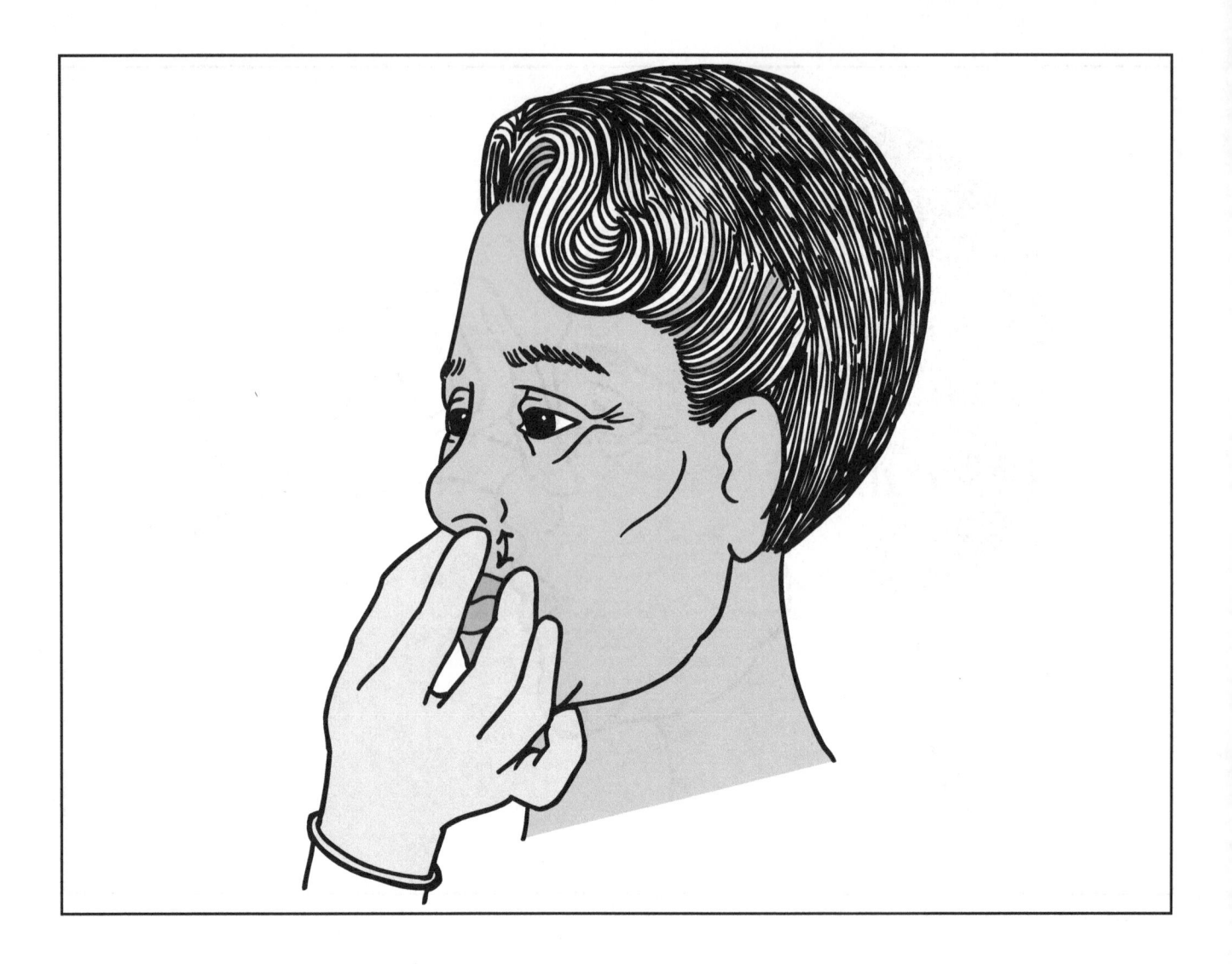

Chapter 12, continued

Pinch the flesh under the nose vertically with the thumb and index finger. Then twist from side to side. Repeat the twisting motion 3 times. Breathe in deeply, holding the breath at first and then exhale effortlessly.

Benefit

- provides acupressure stimulation to pressure points that regulate energy flow for digestive tract (aids in constipation, indigestion, relief of flatulence)

Chapter 13:
Ears, Eyes, and Brow Exercises

Attending to the Musculature of the Ears

Over 100 body regulating points are in the ears. Stretching the ear relieves tension in the head, especially the temporomandibular joint and surrounding musculature. Light massage of the ear contributes to good energy flow and corresponding alertness in the individual.

Both ears can be moved at the same time or you can do one ear at a time.

1. Brush the ear forward, flattening it against the head. Repeat the motion 5 times.

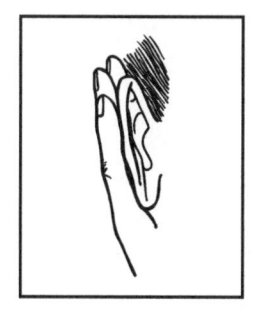

2. Gently pull the earlobe down with the index finger and thumb.

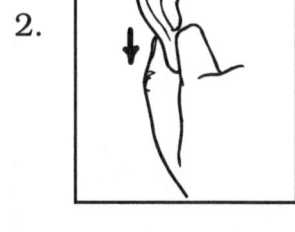

3. Trace the spiral curve of the ear with an index finger. Gently rub all around the spiral channel 2 to 3 times.

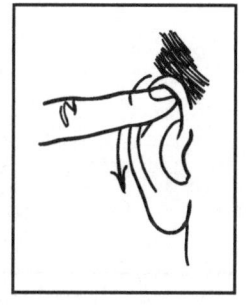

4. Gently grab the ridge of the ear close to the ear canal with index finger and thumb. Squeeze inner ridge of earlobe.

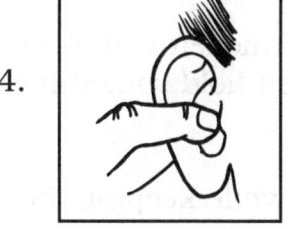

Note: After performing these exercises, ask the client, "Do you feel any pain or tension elsewhere in your head, face, or neck?" If the client indicates the back of the neck, for example, continue with interventions that address that area. Releasing blockages, tension, and imbalances in the head, face, oral cavity, and neck may allow the client better control of fine motor musculature for speech, voicing, and swallowing.

The Oral-Facial Therapy Exercise Book
2021 Edition

Eye Socket Stretch

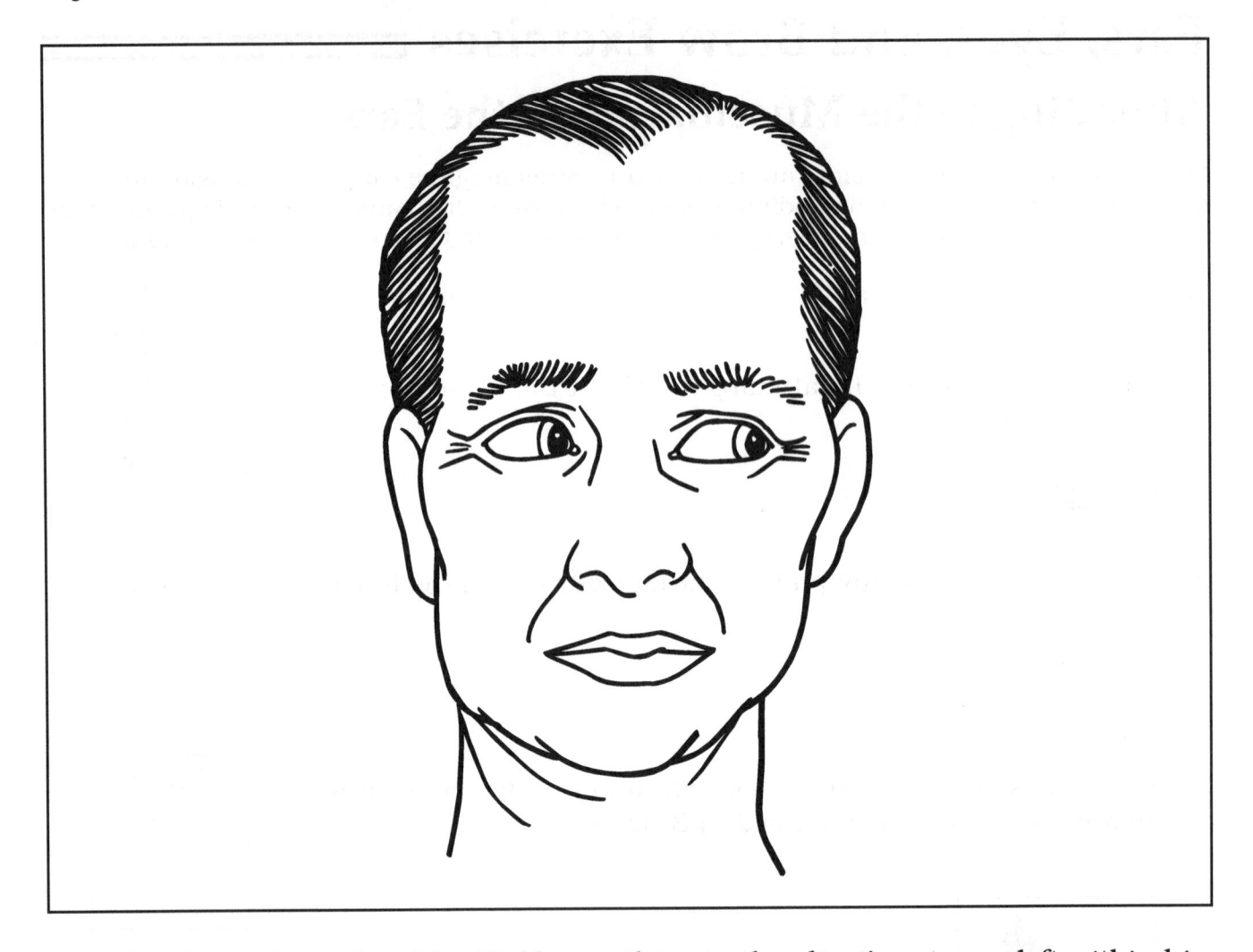

Chapter 13, continued

Keep head upright and stable. Hold something to the client's extreme left within his visual range. Have the client look at it, moving his eyes only. Then hold something on the client's right side. Repeat on each side.

Then have the client look up and then down as much as possible while keeping the head stable.

Remind the client to breathe during this exercise.

Benefit

○ stretches the entire ocular and sinus area

Forehead Massage

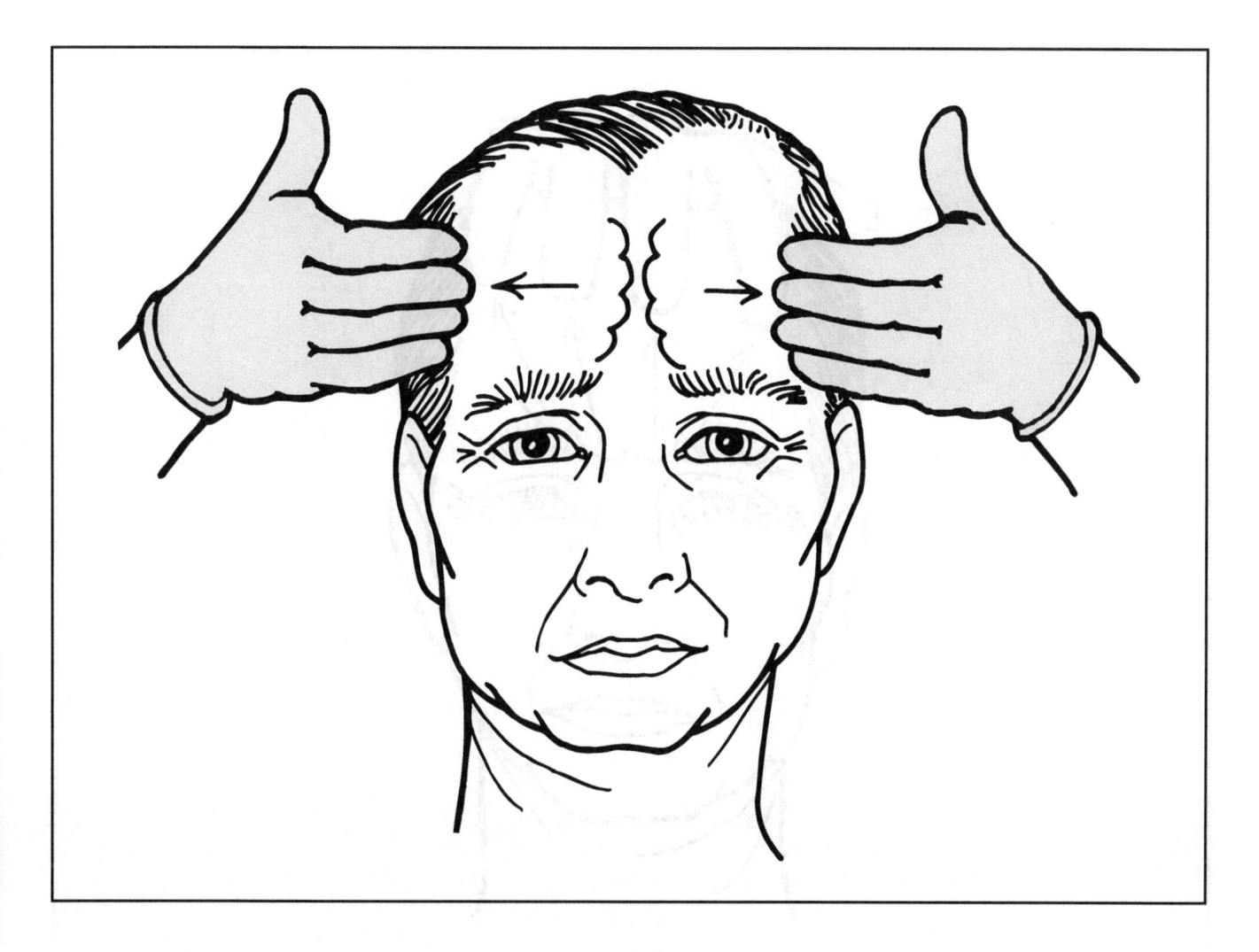

Chapter 13, continued

Put all fingers over eyebrows, touching vertically. Apply gentle pressure and pull hands outward toward temples, straight across sustaining light pressure with fingertips. Repeat.

Benefits

- relaxes and tones head musculature
- reduces muscular strain associated with squinting
- reduces temple pain associated with headaches

Brow and Forehead Stretch

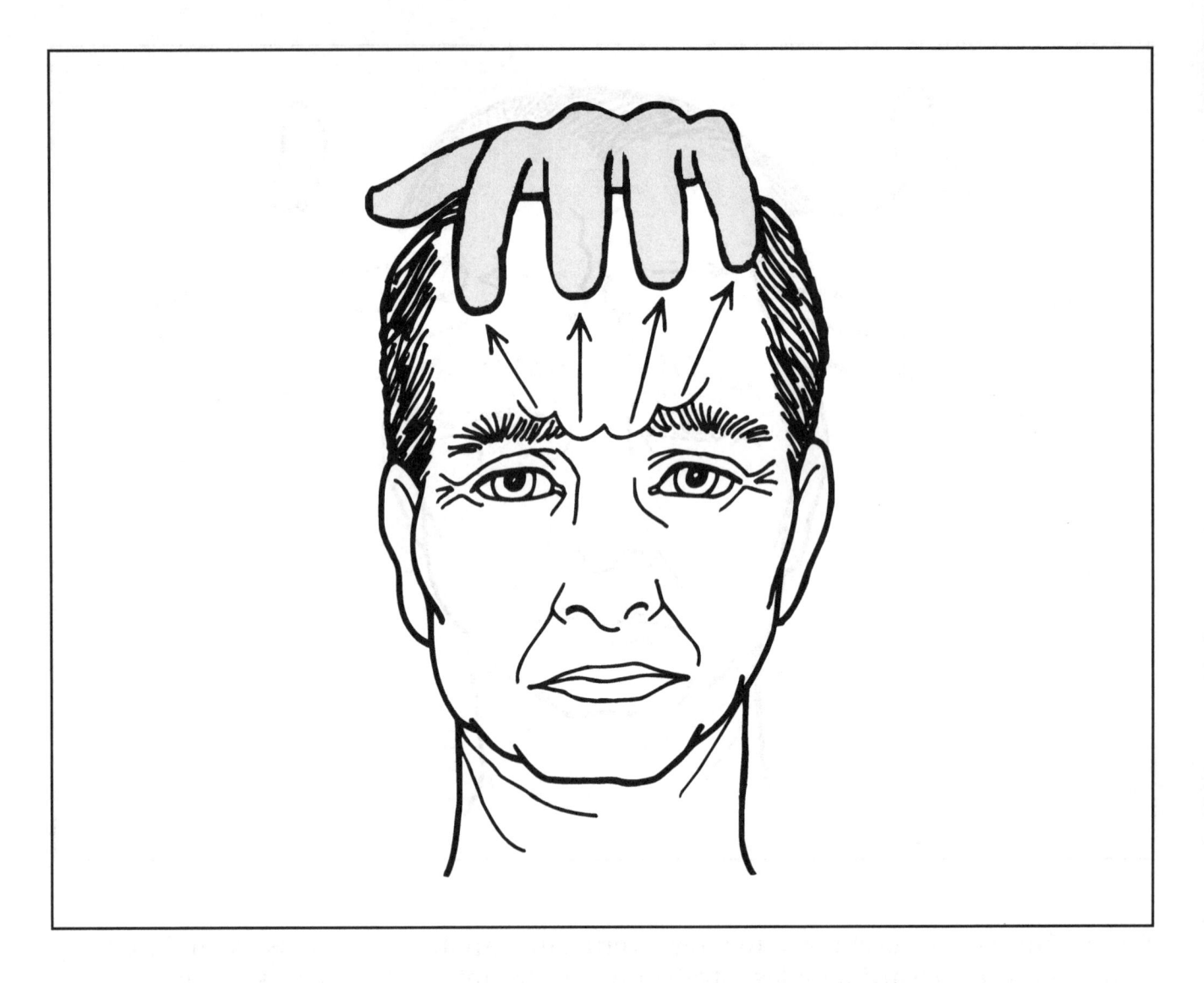

Chapter 13, continued

Place fingertips between eyes and above eyebrows with fingers close together. Move fingers upward, fanning fingers with gentle steady pressure into and through hairline. Repeat. Relax all facial musculature.

Benefits

- stretches and tones brow and forehead
- reduces eye and forehead strain, frowning, and squinting

Assessments, Evaluations, and Forms

The evaluations and forms on the following pages will aid you in evaluating and assisting clients with oral-facial disorders.

- Referral Sheet
- Request for Release of Medical Records
- Oral-Facial Swallowing Evaluation and Rating Scale
- Oral-Facial Function Evaluation
- Visual Facial Charting
- Client Care Plan
- Neurological Daily Status Update
- Speech-Language Pathology Status Update
- Phonation Chart
- Oral Motor Exercise Chart - Lips
- Oral Motor Exercise Chart - Tongue

Referral Sheet

Referral Date _____ Agency _____

Client Name _____ Date of Birth _____

Client Number _____ Age _____

Address _____

Start of Care _____

Physician _____ Phone _____

Caregiver/Contact _____

Primary Diagnosis _____

Secondary Diagnosis _____

Medications _____
_____

Are client and family aware of diagnosis? _____

Physical Limitations _____

Food Allergies _____

Reports of Other Testing _____
_____

Other Services the Client Is Receiving _____
_____

Clinician's Name _____

Date and Time of Scheduled Evaluation _____

Notes _____
_____

Request for Release of Medical Records

To _____
Physician

_____
Street Address

_____
City   State   Zip

I hereby request that my medical records be released to:

_____
Physician

_____
Street Address

_____
City   State   Zip

_____
Client (Print name)

_____
Client Signature

_____
Street Address

_____
City   State   Zip

_____
Birthdate   Social Security Number

Oral-Facial Swallowing Evaluation and Rating Scale

Client Name _____ Evaluation Date _____

Date of Birth _____ Clinician _____

Primary Diagnosis _____ Date of Onset _____

Secondary Diagnosis _____ Date of Onset _____

Medical History (past/present): _____
_____
_____

Medication (past/present): _____
_____

Allergies (past/present): _____
_____

Surgeries or Medical Intervention _____
_____
_____
_____
_____
_____

Respiratory status ☐ respiratory therapy
 ☐ tracheostomy tube status (history of pneumonia) _____

General physical status (e.g., weak, dehydrated) _____
_____
_____
_____
_____

The Oral-Facial Therapy Exercise Book
2021 Edition

Orientation Test to Determine Accurate Yes/No Responses

Check all that apply.

- ❏ Are you a man or a woman?
- ❏ Are you tall?
- ❏ Are you eating?
- ❏ Are you standing?
- ❏ Is it nighttime?
- ❏ Is your name Bob?
- ❏ Are you wearing gloves?
- ❏ Do you have a hand?
- ❏ Is there a glass on the table?
- ❏ Look to the left. Is there a glass there? (Place glass on left or right and ask yes/no question.)

____/10 Total Correct   ____%   Average response time per question _____

Comments: _____
_____

Sensory Processing

Check all that apply.

- ❏ fearful of movements (e.g., taking a drive in the car, movement in the wheelchair)
- ❏ avoids crowded areas (e.g., mall, gym, grocery store, theater)
- ❏ avoids textures (e.g., sticky, rough, textured, wet, cold)
- ❏ overly sensitive to sounds, dislikes loud sounds
- ❏ distractible/impulsive/hyperactive
- ❏ tends to repeat
- ❏ marked mood variations: outburst, tantrums, silliness
- ❏ self-stimulatory behavior (e.g., hitting head, scratching) List: _____
_____

The Oral-Facial Therapy Exercise Book
2021 Edition

Cognitive Function

Check all that apply.

- ☐ alert
- ☐ follows commands
- ☐ lethargic
- ☐ disoriented
- ☐ aphasic
- ☐ dysarthric
- ☐ agitated
- ☐ apraxic

Cognitive Function: _____

_____

Memory/Attention: _____

_____

Vision: _____

Hearing: _____

Other: _____

Gross Motor/Fine Motor Skills

Resting Posture: _____

Feeding Posture: _____

Food Transfer Skills: _____

Handedness: _____

Assisted by: _____

Adaptive Feeding Equipment: _____

Description of Swallowing

Current Nutritional Inventory   Date of Transfer to Each

- ☐ oral   _____
- ☐ nasogastric tube   _____
- ☐ intravenous   _____
- ☐ gastrostomy   _____
- ☐ other _____   _____

Weight ____ (gain or loss)   Hydration needs: _____

Special Dietary Concerns: (e.g., sodium, albumin, total protein levels, sugar, potassium)

_____

_____

Oral Transit Time and Motion of Tongue: _____

Description of Swallowing, continued

Swallow Reflex:

❑ immediate to under one second
❑ under two seconds
❑ several second delay
❑ double swallow observed before bolus cleared

Reported time taken for a typical meal: _____

Check all that apply during or after swallowing:

❑ choking   ❑ watery eyes
❑ increase in heart rate   ❑ nasal regurgitation
❑ coughing   ❑ taste change
❑ appetite change   ❑ dry mouth
❑ heartburn   ❑ pain
❑ difficulty catching breath   ❑ increased congestion
❑ change in ability to smell   ❑ voice change (e.g., wet voice quality)
❑ mouth odor   ❑ drooling or spillage of food or liquid
❑ pocketing of food between the   ❑ sensation of food getting "stuck"
   cheek and gum or anywhere else

Check all techniques client currently uses to compensate:

❑ double swallow   ❑ separates consistencies
❑ head down   ❑ decreases bolus size
❑ turns head toward weaker side   ❑ slows feeding
❑ coughs   ❑ expectorates
❑ holds breath

List tolerances with food consistencies and food preferences (as observed by family, caregivers, nursing staff, and food testing)

_____

_____

Describe type and amount of food and liquid consumed in 48-hour period (include number of meals)

_____

_____

The Oral-Facial Therapy Exercise Book
2021 Edition

Description of Swallowing, continued

Describe changes in oral sensation (change in temperature awareness, change in taste awareness)
_____
_____

- ❏ no swallowing difficulties observed and/or reported
- ❏ possible swallowing difficulties observed and/or reported
- ❏ swallowing difficulties observed and/or reported

Notes: _____
_____

Oral-Facial Structure Examination (Check if structure is present and within normal limits. Note any changes, abnormalities, prosthesis and if oral-facial structure or deviation is possibly contributing to dysphagia)

- ❏ lips _____
- ❏ teeth _____
- ❏ tongue _____
- ❏ floor of mouth _____
- ❏ cheeks _____
- ❏ faucial arches _____
- ❏ tonsils _____
- ❏ hard palate _____
- ❏ soft palate _____
- ❏ uvula _____
- ❏ posterior pharyngeal wall _____
- ❏ maxilla _____
- ❏ mandible _____

Oral-Facial Function Evaluation

Rating Scale Key (Circle more than one number if needed.)

1 - Appropriate range of motion, strength of musculature, and rate
2 - Slowed rate (range of motion and tone normal)
3 - Reduced range of motion
4 - Abnormal or atypical movement patterns
5 - Mild to moderate muscle weakness
6 - Severe muscle weakness
7 - Paresis
NA - Not applicable or not age appropriate

Musculature	Rating Normal————Paresis	Observations (Note asymmetry, hypotonicity, hypertonicity, or compensating musculature)

Lip Closure
   resting position
   bilabial repetition
   during oral phase/swallow
Lateralization
Purse
	
	1 2 3 4 5 6 7 NA
	1 2 3 4 5 6 7 NA
	1 2 3 4 5 6 7 NA
	1 2 3 4 5 6 7 NA
	1 2 3 4 5 6 7 NA	

Tongue Elevation of Tip
   slight jaw opening
   wide jaw opening
   sweep front to back on hard to soft palate
   placement during repetition of /ti/
   placement /t/ or /d/ in sentence
     ("I eat at Tammy's house tonight" or "Dig down under the dirt, Diane.")
	
	1 2 3 4 5 6 7 NA
	1 2 3 4 5 6 7 NA
	1 2 3 4 5 6 7 NA
	
	1 2 3 4 5 6 7 NA
	1 2 3 4 5 6 7 NA	

Tongue Elevation of Back
   slight jaw opening
   wide jaw opening
   placement during repetition of /ki/
   placement /k/ or /g/ in sentence
     ("Can I cook corn on the cob, Mickey?" or "Goggles are good for swimming.")
	
	1 2 3 4 5 6 7 NA
	1 2 3 4 5 6 7 NA
	1 2 3 4 5 6 7 NA
	1 2 3 4 5 6 7 NA	

Tongue Retraction Tongue Widening	1 2 3 4 5 6 7 NA 1 2 3 4 5 6 7 NA	

Tongue Lateralization
   front left
   back left
   front right
   back right
   left buccal sweep
   right buccal sweep
	
	1 2 3 4 5 6 7 NA
	1 2 3 4 5 6 7 NA
	1 2 3 4 5 6 7 NA
	1 2 3 4 5 6 7 NA
	1 2 3 4 5 6 7 NA
	1 2 3 4 5 6 7 NA	

Mandible
   left
   right
   open
	
	1 2 3 4 5 6 7 NA
	1 2 3 4 5 6 7 NA
	1 2 3 4 5 6 7 NA	

Neck
   head to left
   head to right
   head down front
	
	1 2 3 4 5 6 7 NA
	1 2 3 4 5 6 7 NA
	1 2 3 4 5 6 7 NA	

Pharyngeal/Gag Reflex (Tell client you are going to gag him/her to note pharyngeal musculature. Describe strong sphincter contraction of pharyngeal wall, elevation of soft palate, bilateral uniform movement, or weakness unilaterally or bilaterally.)

_____

Ability to chew (appropriate, restricted, weak) _____

Ability to cough (on command, estimated strength of cough) _____

_____

Ability to clear throat (on command, estimated strength of throat clear) _____

_____

Phonation (Circle applicable characteristics.)

hoarse	breathy	harsh
glottal fry	diplophonia	tremor
pitch breaks	aphonia	whisper
monotone	hypernasal	hyponasal
pharyngeal fricatives	nares constriction	situational or intermittent
strained	phonation breaks	hard glottal attack
cul-de-sac (obstructed, closed back sound)		

Intelligibility _____

Vocal quality _____

Loudness _____

Pitch _____

Rate _____

Intonation _____

Resonance _____

Maximum phonation time for /a/: ____ seconds (average adult 15-20 seconds)

Maximum phonation time for /i/: ____ seconds (average adult 15-22 seconds)

Check if observed:

- ❏ congestion
- ❏ mouth breathing
- ❏ current upper respiratory infection
- ❏ facial grimacing
- ❏ excessive mucosa/saliva
- ❏ audible inhalations
- ❏ enlarged tonsils/adenoids
- ❏ nasal emission of air
- ❏ neck/laryngeal tension

The Oral-Facial Therapy Exercise Book
2021 Edition

Phonation, continued

Check if reported:

- ❏ habitual throat clearing
- ❏ habitual coughing
- ❏ screaming
- ❏ sound and voice imitations
- ❏ smoking (past or present) _____
- ❏ alcohol consumption (past or present) _____
- ❏ other _____

Interpersonal Considerations (Check if indicated and elaborate.)

- ❏ inappropriate actions or responses
- ❏ poor motivation
- ❏ depression
- ❏ stress
- ❏ denial associated with abilities and recovery
- ❏ anxiety
- ❏ anger
- ❏ lacking listening skills
- ❏ aggressive behavior
- ❏ verbally abusive

Comments _____

Describe living situation (Note how client best communicates or relates to hobbies, interests, favorite TV shows, music, etc.): _____
_____

Impressions: _____
_____
_____

Recommendations: _____
_____

Referrals: _____
_____

_____   _____
Evaluator Signature   Date

_____   _____
Physician Signature   Date

The Oral-Facial Therapy Exercise Book
2021 Edition

Case Management Information

Client Name _____

Age _____ ☐ Male ☐ Female

Diagnosis _____
_____

Phase of Illness ☐ acute ☐ severe
☐ long-standing condition ☐ recent onset

Social/Work/Caretaker/Home Factors _____
_____
_____

Oral-Motor Dysfunction Measure of Severity

☐ mild ☐ moderate ☐ severe

Eating Method/Ability (Check one and explain.)

☐ self ☐ caretaker feeding ☐ nasal tube feeding ☐ gastrointestinal tube feeding
_____
_____

Food Consistency (Check all that apply.)

☐ thin liquids ☐ thickened liquids ☐ pureed ☐ mechanical soft
☐ hard foods ☐ all consistencies

Positioning/Postural Information _____
_____

Nutritional Status (Caloric needs being met? Restrictions/additions to diet?)
_____

Dental Status _____

Medications (List all medications.) _____

Location of Intervention

☐ clinic ☐ home ☐ school ☐ nursing home ☐ workplace

Sample Visual Facial Charting (Pre/Post Therapeutic Intervention)

Client Name _____ Evaluation Date _____

Diagnosis *right side weakness and left side compensating tension* _____

○ Initial Evaluation   ○ Re-evaluation

(Mark as if you're looking directly at the client.)

R   **L**

loss of peripheral vision

Key
- X . . . . . hypertonic (**tense**)
- blank . . . normal
- P . . . . . pain
- lightly shaded . . . . . hypotonic (**flaccid**)
- darkly shaded . . . . . paresis
- O→ . . . . (See notes to side of diagram.)

_____   _____
Suggested Re-evaluation Date   Evaluator

The Oral-Facial Therapy Exercise Book
2021 Edition   Copyright © 2021

Visual Facial Charting (Pre/Post Therapeutic Intervention)

Client Name _____   Evaluation Date _____

Diagnosis _____

○ Initial Evaluation   ○ Re-evaluation

(Mark as if you're looking directly at the client.)

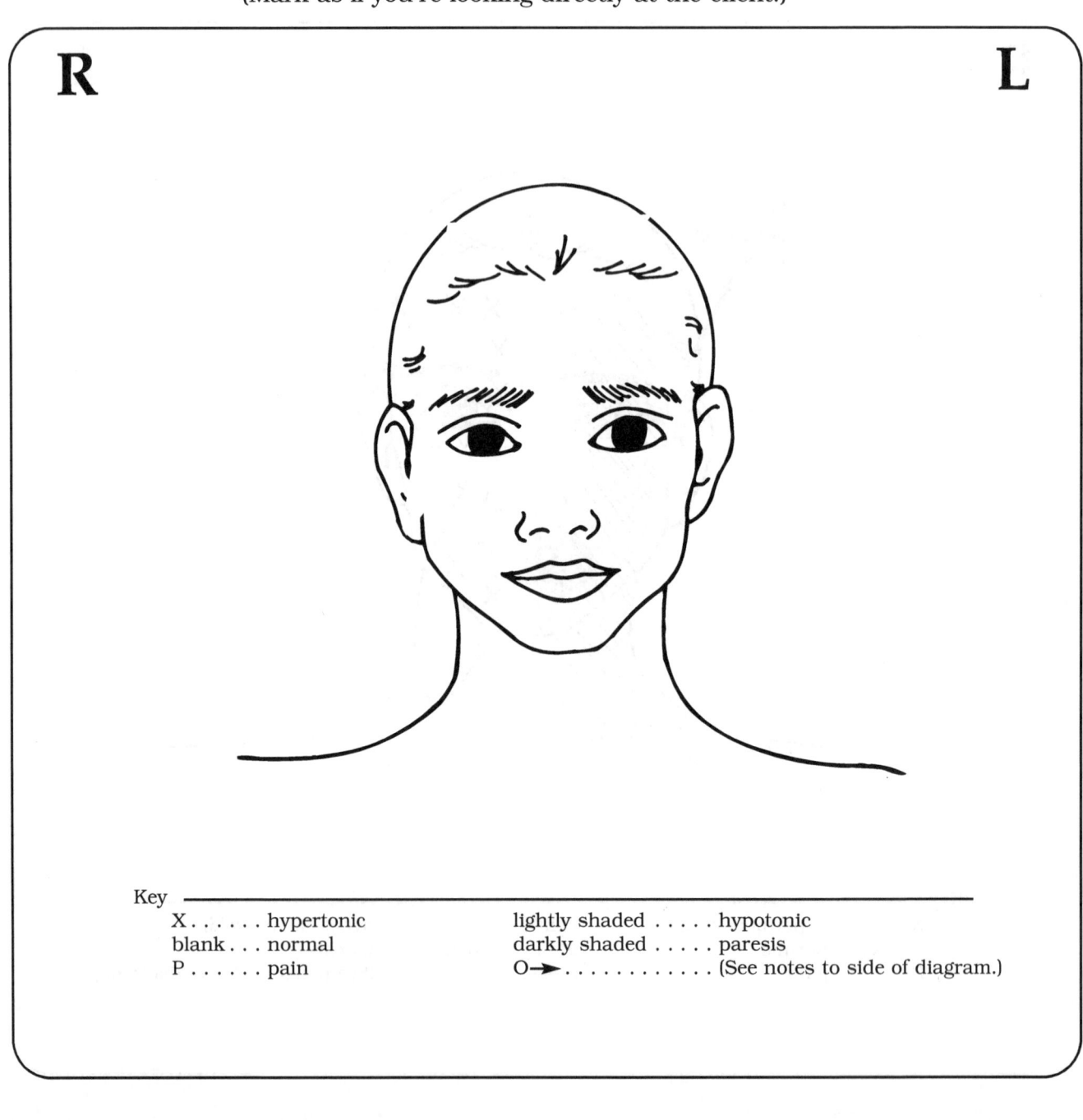

R   **L**

Key
- X . . . . . . hypertonic
- blank . . . normal
- P . . . . . . pain
- lightly shaded . . . . . hypotonic
- darkly shaded . . . . . paresis
- O→ . . . . (See notes to side of diagram.)

_____   _____
Suggested Re-evaluation Date   Evaluator

The Oral-Facial Therapy Exercise Book
2021 Edition   Copyright © 2021

Client Care Plan

Client Name _____ Start of Care _____

Client Number _____ Discharge _____

Clinician _____

Date	Problem	Goal	Intervention Strategy	Date Achieved	Updated Information

The Oral-Facial Therapy Exercise Book
2021 Edition

Neurological Daily Status Update

Client _____

		Time																			
		Date																			
		Initials																			
Nutrition Intake Method	Oral																				
	PEG tube																				
	N-G tube																				
	Combination																				
Food Consistency Type	Liquids																				
	Pureed																				
	Mechanical soft																				
	Hard foods																				
Rancho Levels of Cognitive Functioning*	No response																				
	Generalized response																				
	Localized response																				
	Confused-Agitated																				
	Confused-Inappropriate																				
	Confused-Appropriate																				
	Automatic-Appropriate																				
	Purposeful-Appropriate																				

* See Appendix A, page 243.

The Oral-Facial Therapy Exercise Book
2021 Edition

Neurological Daily Status Update, *continued*

Client _____

Time		
Date		
Initials		
Will Arouse To	Name	
	Shaking	
	Pain	
	Olfactory stimulation	
	Tactile stimulation	
	Loud noise	
	Other	
	None	
Speech	Articulate	
	Dysarthric	
	Apraxic	
	Telegraphic	
	Dysfluent	
	None	

The Oral-Facial Therapy Exercise Book
2021 Edition

Copyright © 2021

Neurological Daily Status Update, *continued*

Client _____

Time		
Date		
Initials		
Ability to Move	Right arm	
	Left arm	
	Right leg	
	Left leg	
	Mouth	
	Tongue	
	Eye opening	
	Head nod	

Speech-Language Pathology Status Update

Client Name _____ Date of Birth _____

Physician _____ Client Number _____

Start of Care _____ Number of Sessions _____

Diagnosis _____

- ❏ Admit
- ❏ Phone Correspondence
- ❏ Biweekly Update
- ❏ Monthly Update
- ❏ Discharge

Notes: _____

_____

_____

_____

_____

_____

_____

_____

_____

_____

_____

_____

_____   _____
        Speech-Language Pathologist   Date

Copies to: _____

_____

_____

The Oral-Facial Therapy Exercise Book

Sample Phonation Chart

Name _____   Start of Care _____

Diagnosis _*vocal strain*_ _____   Physician _____

Clinician _____   Exercise _*Yawn-Sigh*_ _____

Goal _*client will produce /ʌ/ after Yawn-Sigh to reduce hard onset*_ _____

Date	4/22	4/24	4/26							
No. Trials	10	10	10							
Target	VQ	VQ	VQ							
Assistance	C	C	C							
Placement	V	V	V							
Setting	T	T	T							

Hyperadduction
Vocal Strain
Strong

+7
+6
+5
+4   +4
+3   +3
+2
+1   +1

Optimal Voice   0
-1
-2
-3
-4
-5

Hypoadduction
Aphonia
Weak

-6
-7

Target
VQ – vocal quality
VI – vocal intensity
LM – laryngeal musculature
FM – facial musculature

Assistance
M – modeled
C – cued
MT – monitored
I – independent

Placement
V – vowel
W – word
P – phrase
S – sentence
R – reading
RP – role play
CV – conversation

Setting
T – therapy
H – home

The Oral-Facial Therapy Exercise Book
2021 Edition

Phonation Chart

Name _____ Start of Care _____

Diagnosis _____ Physician _____

Clinician _____ Exercise _____

Goal _____

Date									
No. Trials									
Target									
Assistance									
Placement									
Setting									

Hyperadduction
Vocal Strain
Strong

+7
+6
+5
+4
+3
+2
+1

Optimal Voice 0

-1
-2
-3
-4
-5

Hypoadduction
Aphonia
Weak

-6
-7

Target	**Assistance**	**Placement**		**Setting**
VQ – vocal quality	M – modeled	V – vowel	R – reading	T – therapy
VI – vocal intensity	C – cued	W – word	RP – role play	H – home
LM – laryngeal musculature	MT – monitored	P – phrase	CV – conversation	
FM – facial musculature	I – independent	S – sentence		

The Oral-Facial Therapy Exercise Book
2021 Edition   177   Copyright © 2021

Oral-Motor Exercise Chart - Lips

Client _____

Target:
LC - lip closure
LR - lip retraction
LP - lip purse
LPR - lip protrude

Assistance:
F - full assistance
C - cued
I - independent

P - partial assistance
M - monitored

Setting: T - therapy
H - home

Date										
No. Trials										
Target										
Assistance										
Setting										

+10 — Strong

+5 — Medium

0 — Weak or No Movement

Relative Strength

The Oral-Facial Therapy Exercise Book
2021 Edition

Copyright © 2021

Oral-Motor Exercise Chart - Tongue

Client _____

Target: TE - tongue extension
TR - tongue retraction
TW - tongue widening

BF - bowl formation
TP - tip raising
TN - tongue narrowing

Assistance: C - cued
I - independent

Setting: T - therapy
H - home

Date										
No. Trials										
Target										
Assistance										
Setting										

+10 — Strong

+5 — Medium

0 — Weak or No Movement

Relative Strength

The Oral-Facial Therapy Exercise Book
2021 Edition

179

Copyright © 2021

Rancho Levels of Cognitive Functioning

It is imperative to know the cognitive functioning level of the client to determine the type of therapeutic intervention. The following scale can augment observation and testing in determining cognitive functioning and initiation of therapeutic intervention.

Level One: No Response

- No response to pain, touch, sound, or sight
- Appears to be in a deep sleep

Level Two: Generalized Response

- Responses inconsistent independent of stimuli presented
- Delayed responses characterized by gross body movements and/or vocalizations
- Response to deep pain

Level Three: Localized Response

- Responses are directly related to stimulus presented. For example, turning head toward sound.
- Follows commands inconsistently in delayed manner
- Shows vague body awareness such as pulling at N-G tube or resisting restraints
- Shows a bias by responding to one individual over another, such as family, but not clinician

Level Four: Confused-Agitated

- Alert, very active, aggressive, or bizarre behaviors
- Performs motor activities, but behavior is non-purposeful
- Extremely short attention span
- Unaware of present events and responds to past events
- Unable to perform hygiene or self-care

Level Five: Confused-Inappropriate

- Gross attention to environment
- Highly distractible
- Requires continual redirection
- Difficulty learning new tasks
- Agitated by too much stimulation
- May engage in social conversation, but with inappropriate verbalizations
- Responds to simple command fairly consistently
- Performs self-care with assistance
- Inappropriate use of objects without outside direction

Level Six: Confused-Appropriate

- Goal directed behavior with external output
- Able to tolerate unpleasant stimuli (e.g., N-G tube)
- Inconsistent orientation to time and place
- Retention span/recent memory impaired
- Begins to recall past
- Consistently follows simple directions
- Goal-directed behavior with assistance

Level Seven: Automatic-Appropriate

- Performs daily routine in highly familiar environment in a non-confused but automatic robot-like manner
- Skills noticeably deteriorate in unfamiliar environment
- Lacks realistic planning for own future
- Shows increased awareness of self, family, food, and environment
- Unable to drive a car
- Pre-vocational skill assessment indicated at this point

Level Eight: Purposeful and Appropriate

- Alert and able to integrate past, recent, and present events
- Requires no supervision and is independent based on physical capabilities
- Social, emotional, and intellectual abilities may be reduced, but client is functional for society

Reprinted by permission from Hagen, C., Malkmus, D., and Durham, P. The Rancho Los Amigos Hospital, Inc. Downey, CA: Professional Staff Association.

Standardized Speech Samples

It is helpful to have a standardized speech sample. Have the individual read the entire first paragraph but do not measure the first and last sentences. The remaining four sentences provide a 55-word (76-syllable) sample. The entire Rainbow Passage is included for further sample material.

The Rainbow Passage

When sunlight strikes raindrops in the air, they act like a prism and form a rainbow. The rainbow is a division of white light into many beautiful colors. These take the shape of a long round arch, with its path high above, and its two ends apparently beyond the horizon. There is, according to legend, a boiling pot of gold at one end. People look but no one ever finds it. When a man looks for something beyond his reach, his friends say he is looking for the pot of gold at the end of the rainbow.

Throughout the centuries men have explained the rainbow in various ways. Some have accepted it as a miracle without physical explanation. To the Hebrews it was a token that there would be no more universal floods.

The Greeks used to imagine that it was a sign from the gods to foretell war or heavy rain. The Norsemen considered the rainbow as a bridge over which the gods passed from the earth to their home in the sky. Other men have tried to explain the phenomenon physically. Aristotle thought that the rainbow was caused by reflection of the sun's rays by the rain. Since then physicists have found that it is not the reflection, but refraction by the raindrops which causes the rainbow. Many complicated ideas about the rainbow have been formed. The difference in the rainbow depends considerably upon the size of the water drops, and the width of the colored band increases as the size of the drops increases.

The actual primary rainbow observed is said to be the effect of superposition of a number of bows. If the red of the second bow falls upon the green of the first, the result is to give a bow with an abnormally wide yellow band, since red and green light when mixed form yellow. This is a very common type of bow, one showing mainly red and yellow, with little or no green or blue.

Grandfather Passage

You wish to know all about my grandfather. Well, he is nearly 93 years old, yet he still thinks as swiftly as ever. He dresses himself in an old black frock coat, usually several buttons missing. A long beard clings to his chin, giving those who observe him a pronounced feeling of the utmost respect. When he speaks, his voice is just a bit cracked and quivers a bit. Twice each day he plays skillfully and with zest upon a small organ. Except in the winter when the snow or ice prevents, he slowly takes a short walk in the open air each day. We have often urged him to walk more and smoke less, but he always answers, "Banana oil!" Grandfather likes to be modern in his language.

The Wish

May you always find serenity and tranquility in a world you may not understand.

May the pain you have known and the conflict you have experienced give you the strength to walk through life facing each new situation with courage and optimism. Always know that those who love and understand will be there, even when you feel most alone. May you discover enough goodness in others to believe in a world of peace. May a kind word, a reassuring touch, and a warm smile be yours every day of your life, and may you give these gifts as well as receive them. Remember the sunshine when the storm seems unending. Teach love to those who know hate and let that love embrace you as you go into the world.

May the teachings of those you admire become part of you so that you may call upon them. Remember that those whose lives you have touched and who have touched yours are always a part of you, even if the encounters were less than you would have wished. It is the content of the encounter that is more important than the form. May you not become too concerned with material matters, but instead place immeasurable value on the goodness in your heart. Find time in each day to see beauty and love in the world around you.

Realize that each person has limitless abilities, but each of us is different in our own way. What you may feel you lack in one regard may be more than compensated for in another. What you feel you lack in the present may become one of your strengths in the future. May you see your future as one filled with promise and possibility. Learn to view everything as a worthwhile experience. May you find enough inner strength to determine your own worth by yourself, and not be dependent on another's judgment of your accomplishments.

May you always feel loved.

Affirmation for Composure and Harmony

Composed and peaceful, I enter a meaningful and productive day. In the course of the day beginning, I shall welcome difficulties with composure, remembering that hardships are there to challenge my fortitude and develop my strength. I will make everyone I meet today a better person; every act of mine will be a sign of peace and of the voice of nature.

(de Langre 1989)

Front View of Muscles

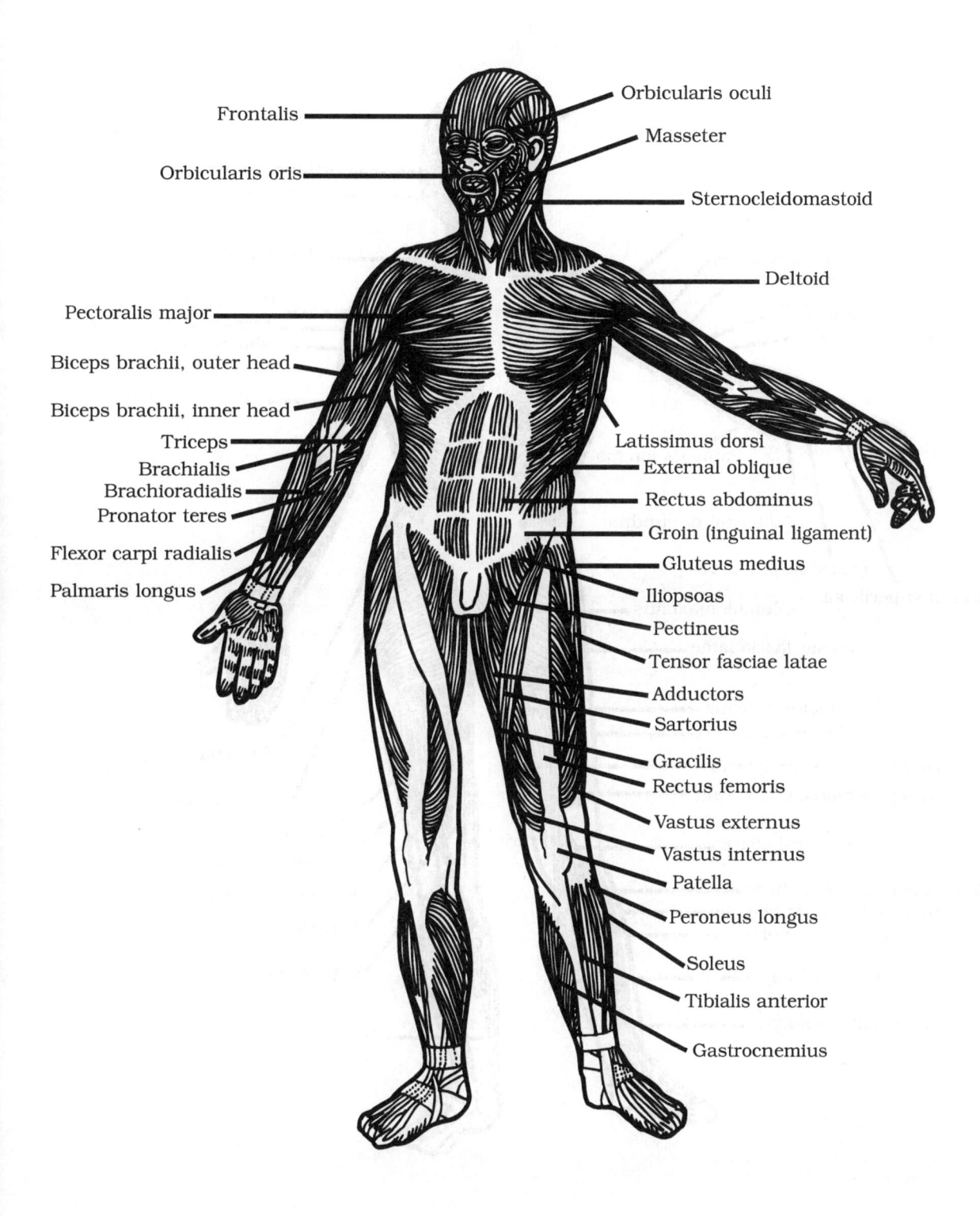

- Frontalis
- Orbicularis oris
- Pectoralis major
- Biceps brachii, outer head
- Biceps brachii, inner head
- Triceps
- Brachialis
- Brachioradialis
- Pronator teres
- Flexor carpi radialis
- Palmaris longus
- Orbicularis oculi
- Masseter
- Sternocleidomastoid
- Deltoid
- Latissimus dorsi
- External oblique
- Rectus abdominus
- Groin (inguinal ligament)
- Gluteus medius
- Iliopsoas
- Pectineus
- Tensor fasciae latae
- Adductors
- Sartorius
- Gracilis
- Rectus femoris
- Vastus externus
- Vastus internus
- Patella
- Peroneus longus
- Soleus
- Tibialis anterior
- Gastrocnemius

Back View of Muscles

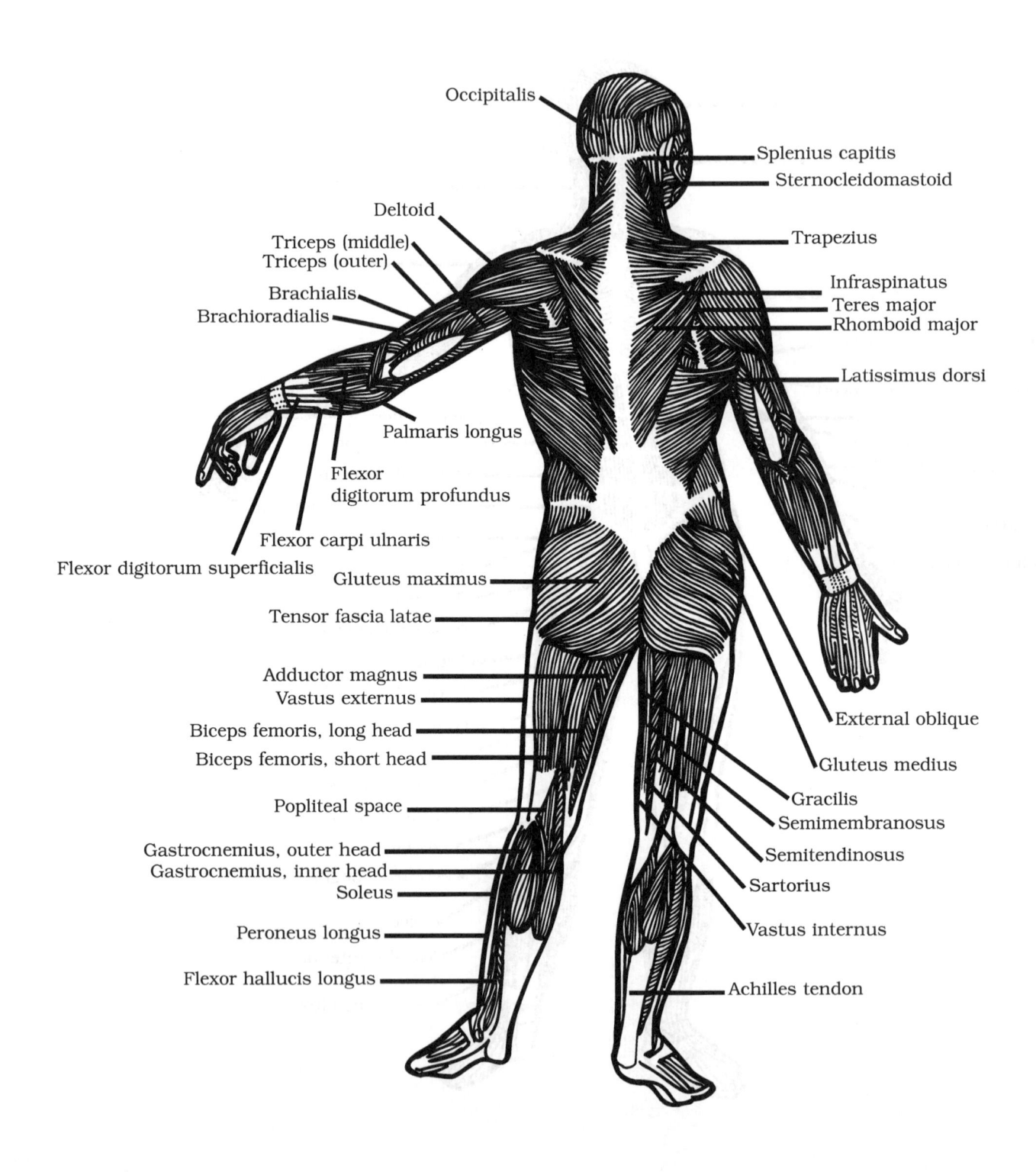

References

Abbott, V. and Brignoni, R. "Dysphagia Team Intervention: Evaluation Through Outcome." Seminar sponsored by Geriatric Research, Education, and Clinical Center, and the Veterans Affairs Medical Center.

Ad-Hoc Committee on Labial-Lingual Posturing Function (ASHA). "The Role of the Speech-Language Pathologist in Assessment and Management of Oral Myofunctional Disorders." *ASHA Supplement #5*, p. 7.

Bahr, D. C. *Oral-Motor Assessment and Treatment: Ages and Stages.* Needham Heights, MA: Allyn and Bacon Publishing.

Barnes, J. F. *Myofascial Release I*, Seminar Workbook. *www.myofascialrelease.com*

Black, J. W. and Ausherman, M. *The Vocabulary of College Students in Classroom Speeches.* Columbus, OH: Bureau of Educational Research, Ohio State University.

Blasco, P. et al. *Management of Saliva Overflow.* (Internet Publication) http://ins.airweb.net/management.htm

Boone, D. *The Voice and Voice Therapy.* Englewood Cliffs, NJ: Prentice-Hall.

Burns, D. *The Feeling Good Handbook.* NYC: William Morrow and Company. Cohen, K.

The Way of Qigong: The Art and Science of Chinese Energy Healing. NYC: Ballantine Books.

Copeland, M. E. *The Worry Control Workbook.* Oakland, CA: New Harbinger Publications, Inc.

Daniels, L. and Worthingham, C. *Muscle Testing.* Philadelphia, PA: W.B. Saunders Company.

de Langre, J. *Do-in 2. The Ancient Art of Rejuvenation Through Self-Massage.* Magalia, CA: Happiness Press.

Dworkin, J. P. *Motor Speech Disorders: A Treatment Guide.* St. Louis, MO: Mosby-Year Book, Inc.

Fairbanks, G. *Voice and Articulation Drillbook.* NYC: Harper and Row.

Ferrin, M. (instructor). "Pediatric Occupational Therapy Course." Palm Beach Community College, Lakeworth, FL.

Gach, M. R. *Acupressure's Potent Points: A Guide to Self-Care for Common Ailments.* NYC: Bantam Doubleday, Dell Publishing Group.

References, continued

Gangale, D. "Acupressure Techniques for Speech Pathologists." (On-line course certified by the American Speech-Language-Hearing Association for Continuing Education Units) *Speechpaths.com*, Professional Marketing Seminars, Newport, CA.

Gangale, D. "Swallowing and the Parkinsonian." *American Parkinsonian Association, Inc., Educational Supplement #2.*

Glanz, M. et al. "Functional Electrostimulation in Post Stroke Rehabilitation: A Meta-Analysis of the Randomized Controlled Trials." *Archives of Physical Medicine and Rehabilitation*, Vol. 77, pp. 549-553.

Howard, P. J. *Owner's Manual for the Brain.* Marietta, GA: Bard Press.

Kagel, M. "Adult Dysphagia Seminar." Presented by Crozer-Chester Medical Center. Communication Symposia, Tampa, FL.

Kenyon, J. *Acupressure Techniques: A Self-Help Guide.* Rochester, VT: Inner Traditions International, Ltd.

Koufman, J. A. "Laryngopharyngeal Reflux and Voice Disorders." *The Visible Voice*, a newsletter published by the Center for Voice Disorders at Wake Forest University, Vol. 3, pp 2-7. *www.bgsm.edu/voice/reflux_voice.html*

Krieger, D. *The Therapeutic Touch: How to Use Your Hands to Help or Heal.* NYC: Simon & Schuster.

Langley, J. *Working with Swallowing Disorders.* Great Britain: Winslow Press.

Lindaman, S. L. "Treatment Techniques for Adult Neurological Dysphagic Patients." Seminar sponsored by the Rehabilitation Institute of Chicago, Chicago, IL.

Logemann, J. *Evaluation and Treatment of Swallowing Disorders.* San Diego, CA: College Hill Press.

Logemann, J. *Normal Swallowing.* Brochure distributed by Menu Magic in cooperation with the American Speech-Language-Hearing Association.

Marshalla, P. "Oral-Motor Techniques in Articulation Therapy." Seminar presented by Innovative Concepts, Inc., Gainesville, FL.

Mattes, A. *Flexibility: Active and Assisted Stretching.* Sarasota, FL: Mattes.

McClure, V. *Infant Massage: A Handbook for Loving Parents.* New York: Bantam Books.

References, continued

Michels Jelm, J. *Oral-Motor/Feeding Rating Scale.* Tucson, AZ: Communication Skill Builders, Inc., a division of The Psychological Corporation.

Myss, C. *Anatomy of the Spirit: The Seven Stages of Power and Healing.* NYC: Random House, Inc.

Nicolosi, L. et al. *Terminology of Communication Disorders.* Baltimore, MD: Williams and Wilkins.

Orloff, J. *Dr. Judith Orloff's Guide to Intuitive Healing: Five Steps to Physical, Emotional, and Sexual Wellness.* NYC: Random House.

Painter, J. *Deep Bodywork and Personal Development, Harmonizing Our Bodies, Emotions, and Thoughts.* Olympia, WA: Bodymind Books.

Prudden, B. *Pain Erasure, The Bonnie Prudden Way.* NYC: Ballentine.

Swigert, N. B. *The Source for Dysarthria.* East Moline, IL: LinguiSystems, Inc.

Tappen, F. *Healing Massage Techniques: Holistic, Classic, and Emerging Methods.* E. Norwalk, CT: Appleton and Lange, a division of Prentice Hall.

Teeguarden, I. M. *The Joy of Feeling: Bodymind Acupressure.* NYC: Japan Publications/Harper & Row.

White, C. "Nasogastric Intubation-Oral and Perioral Care." *Special Care and Dentistry.* Vol. 4, No. 1, January-February.

Ylvisaker, M. *Head Injury Rehabiliation: Children and Adolescents.* San Diego, CA: College Press.

Made in United States
Troutdale, OR
03/01/2024